COPING
YOUR CERVIC

KAREN EVENNETT graduated from University College London in 1983. She worked in academic publishing before training as a journalist at the London College of Printing in 1986. She now specializes in writing about women's health and relationships and her features appear regularly in the national newspapers and women's magazines *Woman's Own*, *Woman's Realm*, *She*, *Best*, and *Bella*. Karen has written one other book for Sheldon Press, *Coping Successfully with PMS* (1995). She lives in Surrey and is married with one daughter, Coco.

Overcoming Common Problems Series

For a full list of titles please contact
Sheldon Press, Marylebone Road, London NW1 4DU

Overcoming Common Problems Series

Overcoming Common Problems Series

Overcoming Common Problems

COPING WITH
YOUR CERVICAL SMEAR

Karen Evennett

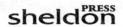

First published in Great Britain in 1996 by
Sheldon Press, SPCK, Marylebone Road, London NW1 4DU

British Library Cataloguing-in-Publication Data
A catalogue record for this book is available from the
British Library

ISBN 0–85969–734–7

Photoset by Deltatype Ltd, Ellesmere Port, Cheshire
Printed in Great Britain
by Biddles Ltd, Guildford and King's Lynn

Contents

Introduction

When Roz moved from Liverpool to Bristol in the 1980s, her new GP informed her that in this health authority cervical smear tests were offered to woman once every five years and not, as she had become used to at her old practice, every three years.

'I told him I thought that was far too long to wait,' Roz says. 'My mother had died of cancer – though not of the cervix – and because cancer was in my family I'd always had the fear that this is what would eventually kill me.'

The doctor said he could understand Roz's anguish, but told her, 'In this area, unless I can give a very good reason for you needing an earlier smear, the lab won't even run the test on it. You would have to pay a private clinic if you wanted a smear before your allotted time comes up.'

When Roz's allotted time eventually did come up, she learned she had abnormal cells classed as CIN 3, the last stage before becoming 'invasive cancer'.

'Three months later, at the age of 34, never having had children, I was admitted to hospital for a hysterectomy,' she says.

On the one hand, Roz considers herself lucky that the cells were still pre-cancerous – had the smear been timed to take place say a year later, she might already have had invasive cancer.

On the other hand, though, Roz cannot help but feel bitter that the test was not run earlier, when she wanted it, and when she would have had the opportunity to receive laser or diathermy treatment, which would have saved her womb and allowed her the chance to one day have children.

The smear test's job is to detect for pre-cancerous changes, which are known to doctors as CIN conditions. CIN 1 is the mildest form of pre-cancer. CIN 3 is the most severe, and while Roz was most unfortunate and very unusual in having to undergo an operation to remove her womb, most women with any stage of CIN can be treated using far less radical techniques. What is more, once the treatment is completed, they are, in most cases, completely free of the cells that, had they been left untreated, could have become cancer. It is for this reason that the smear test is so important to the well-being of women, and it has saved millions of lives.

This book brings together women's stories of smear tests, doctors' attitudes, and the treatments women have endured. And, through their experiences, I hope to make you aware of the choices available to you at each stage of the cervical screening process; and to show you how to get the best treatment you can for yourself.

1

What is a smear test?

When did you last have a cervical smear test? That's a question I've been asking a lot recently, in the course of my research for this book, and very few women have actually been able to give me an accurate answer. 'Oh, a couple of years ago – definitely', one will say. Then, a few seconds later, a puzzled expression creeping over her face, she'll add, 'Or was it the year before that?!' Confusion reigns for a few seconds more and then she'll wave her hand dismissively and say, 'Oh, what does it matter anyway? My doctor's bound to let me know when I need my next one'.

Most of us lead busy lives. We have children's routines, household duties and our own jobs to worry about. A cervical smear often doesn't feature as high on our list of priorities as it should – and it *is* easy to forget when we last had one or when we are due another.

I am as guilty of this as the next woman. When I moved house and changed doctor, my new practice happened to have displayed a large notice asking women if they were due a smear. It occurred to me then that my old medical notes might take many months to reach the new practice so I might as well strike while the iron was hot.

When the doctor asked me how long it had been since my last smear, I had to confess I couldn't remember. All I knew was that it had taken place the same day that some major news story had hit. Neither of us could recall how many years ago this had been, but the doctor agreed it was probably about time I had another one anyway.

Unless you are a particularly organized person, a check-up that takes place every three to five years (for five years is the routine gap left between smears by some health authorites) may easily be overlooked or forgotten.

Today's computerized systems mean that your doctor should send you a reminder when you are due a smear. Occasionally, things do not work out as they should for one reason or another, and you may find that your recall has been missing or delayed. Maybe you have moved house or changed doctor. If you think you are due a smear, you should

3

take yourself along to the doctor for a smear as often as you can.

Who needs a smear?

- Department of Health guidelines recommend that all women between the ages of 20 and 64 should have a cervical smear at least every five years.
- *The British Medical Association Family Health Encyclopedia* recommends that a woman should have a cervical smear within 6 months of first having sexual intercourse, with a second smear 6 to 12 months after that (because of the small chance of missing an abnormality on one smear) and, after that, providing the result is normal, at 3-yearly intervals for the rest of her life.
- Experts at Marie Stopes International recommend that we have smears every year (and although it is not possible for the NHS to provide such a regular service, you have the right to pay for yearly smears if you want them).

There is far too much confusion about the need for regular screening.

One argument against more regular screening is that the trauma of a smear test, the emotional fall-out of a positive result, and the fear of overtreatment or unnecessary treatment outweigh the benefits of regular screening.

For the women whose lives are saved by regular screening, the benefits must win every time. But we are in the hands of doctors, some of whom may even appear to us to have been trained to poo-poo our concerns.

Ten years ago, a friend of mine was studying medicine. We were discussing cervical screening and I said that five years was not, in my opinion, sufficiently regular. He hooted with laughter and said, 'Our lecturer warned us we were likely to come across the occasional loony woman who would demand more regular smears – and he assured us once every five years was quite often enough.'

Now a GP, that medic has quite a different view of our screening guidelines. And he admitted when we were discussing this book that five years really *isn't* good enough, but that it is a decision health authorities have taken on financial grounds. But I wonder whether his old lecturer is still giving tomorrow's doctors the same bad advice he received in medical school.

It has to be pointed out here that in a year in which 1,570,893 cervical smear tests were taken, the majority (1,486,159) were negative. And, of course, if you are one of the many women who go through their entire life never having an abnormal smear, being asked to attend for a test only once every five years really is no problem. However, many women do wish to have smears more often than this, and from the testimonies in this book we can see why more frequent screening really is necessary.

If you want a smear and fear you will not be allowed one because you are not due for one yet, ask your GP anyway. He or she will definitely agree to a smear if there is any reason to suggest you need one: if, for example, you have been bleeding between periods or if you have had an unusual discharge. If you have changed sexual partner frequently or if your partner has had a number of other partners, you also have a good case for asking for more regular smears.

It is also possible that the doctor will simply agree to do the smear on request – you won't know until you ask!

If it is not permissible, and you are concerned, the Women's Nationwide Cancer Control Campaign (see Useful addresses) runs occasional mobile screening units that anyone can attend, free of charge, as well as screening programmes for those working in large companies.

Private cervical smear tests are also available and local clinics will be able to give you a price and further information.

Charitable organizations such as the British Pregnancy Advisory Service (see Useful addresses) also offer smear tests. There is a charge for this service, but, compared to the private sector, it is very low, really no more than you would pay for a haircut.

How is a cervical smear test done?

Your doctor or nurse will ask you to lie on your back with your arms relaxed and your legs bent up and relaxed so that your knees fall open.

The practitioner will then gently insert an instrument called a speculum into your vagina. This shouldn't hurt, but may be painful if you are tense and your vagina is tight.

The speculum holds the vagina open, allowing the practitioner to gently scrape some sample cells from the cervix, which is a small, cylindrical organ, several centimetres in length and less than 2.5 cm in diameter. The cervix comprises the lower part and neck of the womb, and separates the womb from the vagina.

Your doctor or nurse may take these cells using a spatula, or a spatula and a small brush that looks like a delicately bristled mascara brush. The brush allows the practitioner to take a smear from the part of the cervix that the spatula cannot easily reach.

Both the spatula and the brush will then be wiped across a microscope slide so the laboratory can look for any signs of cell changes that may require further investigation.

Why do I need a smear?

The latest figures available for cervical cancer show that, out of a total 4467 cases registered (1988), around 1800 turned out to be fatal. Of the total, 85 per cent of women who develop cervical cancer have never had a smear. The remaining 15 per cent mostly only ever had one smear.

While the smear test does not in itself prevent cancer, it is the only way we have of detecting pre-cancerous changes. If these are treated, cancer will not usually develop. So, by having a smear, and any necessary follow-up treatment, you are, in effect, taking preventative action against cancer. The reasons women may decide *not* to have the test are usually psychological.

- Some women worry that, by volunteering themselves for the test, their partner, friends or relatives will turn on them for having been promiscuous. However, while there is a sexual link with some cancerous and pre-cancerous changes, not *all* cervical cancer has a sexual origin.
- Others fear that the cervical smear test will tell them they have cancer, and they would rather not know, so they avoid being tested. Sadly they are mistaken in thinking the smear's job is to test for cancer. It is to test for pre-cancerous changes. But even in schools, when sixth-form girls are asked, 'Why do you need a smear?', most already believe it is to detect cancer. This is worrying, not

6

only because they are misinformed and will go on being misinformed until someone eventually puts them right, but also because, to many women who do not consider themselves to be in an 'at risk' group for cervical cancer, the mistaken idea that this is what the test is for leads them to believe that it doesn't apply to them and it therefore won't be necessary for them to have the test. As women, we are all at risk of cervical cancer – which is the reason the smear test exists – even though, most of us will not develop the disease.

- There is also the sad group of women who are too embarrassed, nervous or anxious to attend for their smear test.

A clinic manager at Marie Stopes says that women have come to the clinic for smears and have asked for tranquillizers to calm them down. 'One even asked for a general anaesthetic,' she says. At least they turned up. A few are so scared that they don't.

Your first smear ever – be it in your teens, or early twenties – is likely to be the most embarrassing. If it turns out to be a positive experience, you need have no worries in the future. On the other hand, if your experience confirms your worst fears, that the smear test is a grim, embarrassing and painful experience, your nervousness is likely to stay with you.

MARY'S STORY
Mary is 30 now, but she still feels very anxious about cervical smears, and is sure her anxiety stems from her first experience of one when she was 22 years old.

'I have never been so nervous that I have cancelled a smear test – I realize that would be silly, and that I would be putting myself at risk. But I do get extremely nervous. I'm fine prior to the test. But as soon as I am asked to jump up on the doctor's couch, I go into a complete panic. My teeth chatter and I tremble. And the more the doctor tells me to relax, the more tense I become, so that the actual examination is extremely painful.

'What upsets me most of all is the thought of someone other than my partner touching me and putting things inside me. I find it impossible to switch off from the thought of what is happening to me.

'I've asked myself why this should be, and the only answer I can come up with is that my first cervical smear, when I was 22, was a very unpleasant experience.

'My GP was fairly young – possibly unused to smears, I don't know – and he tried to put me at my ease by telling me jokes. Since most of these were crude gynaecological jokes to do with fishy smells, I found they did anything but relax me. I then tensed up so much that the GP had to make several attempts at inserting the speculum, and, although I'm assured this should be a painless procedure, since that first time, it has always been extremely painful for me.'

So how can you make sure that your first smear experience is positive? Or, if you are a mother, that your daughter's smear is not as unpleasant as Mary's?

- Try to make an appointment with a GP or nurse of your choice, if there is a choice at your practice.
- It will help your doctor to relax you if you admit you are anxious.
- Ask him or her to explain what is being done, if you feel it will help you.
- If you are really terrified and want your mother or partner to be present, ask in advance how the GP or nurse would feel about this.

But, whatever you do, don't let anxiety put you off having your smear. It could save your life!

A study by psychologist Alison Bish discovered that even among women who are aware that the test is life-saving, there is reluctance to attend for a smear. She contacted all the women due for a smear test in a one-month period in one London suburb. Most eventually turned up for their screening, but 18 per cent did not. The reasons they gave were that it was embarrassing, distressing, painful and inconvenient.

Britain has the second highest number of deaths from cervical cancer in Europe. Our screening programme is only partly responsible. Women's attitudes to smear tests are also to blame, and I urge you to attend regularly for smears – and to make sure those you love do so, too.

My emphasis on the importance of attending for a smear test may seem contradictory in the light of what I am about to say. It isn't intended to be so.

However ...

Although routine smear tests can identify some changes in the cells of the cervix, the current test, known as the Pap test, hasn't been altered since mass cervical screening started in 1964, and it is not entirely fault-free.

For a start, it relies on human judgement. Cytologists have the task of examining slide after slide, looking for abnormal cells. If they spot any, they have to assess how severe these abnormalities are. And that's basically how the smear is judged.

Most of the work is done by poorly paid laboratory staff and, because it's a tedious job – looking down a microscope – it's very easy to miss abnormal cells. Even the experts acknowledge that current methods of cytology are 10 to 15 per cent inaccurate.

MICHELLE'S STORY

Michelle is 25 years old. Two years ago she discovered she had a cervical abnormality, even though her recent smear test had been returned with a negative result.

'I'd recently had my smear test when I heard that Dr Anne Szarewski, a specialist who works for Marie Stopes and the Margaret Pike Centre, was doing a trial on smokers, to see how smoking affected pre-cancerous changes in the cervix. Since I am, to my shame, a smoker, I thought this would be a great chance to have a really thorough check-up.

'The trial involved going for a colposcopy (a procedure which enables the doctor to take a closer look at the cervix) and also a cervicography (which involves taking photographs of the cervix). And, although my smear test had been negative, these showed a slight abnormality known as CIN 1.

'I was pretty alarmed by this, but Dr Szarewski was reassuring. This was a very small change, and CIN 1 cells often return to normal over time.

'She suggested I now have six-monthly check-ups, and, so far, these have shown that the cells have not deteriorated any further.

Indeed, they appear to be improving. Which is fantastic news.

'What worries me, however, is that my cell change did not register on my original smear test. And, had I waited five years, as many women do, before having another smear, there was the possibility that the cells would have reached an advanced stage of pre-cancer – even though, in actual fact, they did not.'

Michelle is reassured by the fact that she is being looked after, that any further changes will be treated at the earliest opportunity. Not everyone is so lucky.

HAZEL'S STORY

'I've always been conscientious about my smear tests. In 1986, the nurse said she could see some erosion on my cervix. She told me not to worry and that any problems would show up on the smear.

'When the result came back negative, I assumed everything was OK, and I thought no more about it.

'But a few months later, I began to bleed for about half an hour at a time, two or three times a month.

'Since my last smear had shown no abnormalities, the doctor said there was probably nothing to worry about. As a precaution, he referred me to a gynaecologist. I waited several months for the appointment to come through, only to discover I had missed it because my card had been sent to the wrong address. This meant I had to go back on the waiting list.

'In total, I ended up waiting for about five months between seeing my GP and eventually getting to see the gynaecologist.

'It was then that I discovered I had a tumour the size of a ten pence piece, and I needed a course of intensive radiotherapy to remove it.

'I'm still returning to the hospital for annual check-ups. I also have a smear test every year. But I've lost all faith in its reliability.

'Even my GP was astounded when he found out I had cancer. He said he had no idea how bad the Pap test is.'

ANGELA'S STORY

'I laughed out loud when a doctor on television said, "Cervical cancer is the one cancer we can catch. Provided women keep to their three-yearly smears, they'll be OK''.

'I had a clear test in July 1989. But nine months later I began to bleed between periods.

'It was such a small amount, I almost ignored it, but I had to see my doctor about something else anyway. Within a week, I was rushed to hospital for a radical hysterectomy. The cancer was so invasive, the gynaecologist said he could see it even before sending an example for analysis. Yet I had no idea there was anything wrong.

'It will take me a long time to get over the shock.'

Hazel and Angela are understandably cynical about the Pap test. Yet, the doctor Angela saw speaking on the television was correct: in the majority of cases, the smear test *will* pick up abnormalities – and it is for this reason that I stress the importance of attending for your test. Despite its current failings, you are more likely to have your life saved if you are screened regularly than if you are not.

There is hope for the future, however. New tests are in the pipeline.

New tests

The HDA test

One I have reported on in women's magazines is the Quest test (HDA). It offers screening, diagnosis and prognosis in a single test, using a technique that deeply colours the altered genetic material of cancer cells.

It also colours cells in the early stages of cancer that don't show any of the obvious abnormalities required by the present smear test. So current cervical screening would miss them.

The test has been developed by Dr Andrew Sincock of the Galton Laboratory, University College London. He believes it is virtually foolproof as the test is analysed by computer and results will no longer depend on human judgement.

How it works

Screening The HDA (hydrolyzed DNA assay) procedure uses a special stain to colour abnormal genetic material in cells that are pre-cancerous or cancerous. The depth of colour, measured by computer, indicates the severity of cancer-linked abnormality, but no information is yet available regarding the *type* of cancer present, so a secondary approach is needed to analyse the fluorescence rather than the colour resulting from the special stain.

Diagnosis The test diagnoses by using a sophisticated laser microscope to analyse the fluorescent signal. This builds up an image of genetic activity, and results show that patterns of abnormal cancer-linked activity show up clearly when analysed by computer. This suggests it may be possible to provide detailed information about the type of cancer present as a number of clearly recognized patterns of fluorescence have already been identified in different cancers.

Prognosis Information concerning the likely course and outcome of a particular cancer is also a vital component of any cancer test. Early results from the laser analysis also indicate that it may be possible to assess tumour aggression and development.

The Polarprobe test

Another alternative to the smear test of the future is the Polarprobe, a computer-aided machine developed by doctors in Australia. The probe operates on the principle that there are different blood level flows in cancerous and non-cancerous tissue. It is able to pick up these differences via a fat, pencil-shaped probe that is inserted into the vagina and moved across the cervix to check for abnormalities. It is thought to be almost 100 per cent accurate and produces its results within minutes, while the patient is still in the room.

What can you do?

The Government boasts that the number of deaths from cervical cancer is falling in Britain. But, having the second highest death rate in Europe from the disease is nothing to be proud of.

- Do attend your routine smear tests – the current test is still reliable for the majority of women.
- The most common type of cervical cancer occurs only in sexually active women and it's almost certainly linked to some sexually

transmitted organism. You will protect yourself against the disease if your partner always uses a condom during intercourse.

- You should always make an appointment to see your GP about any unusual bleeding, no matter how scant it is, and never feel that you're wasting your doctor's time.
- Do not be alarmed if your smear comes back with an abnormal result. As we will see in the next chapter, your diagnosis now means you are one of the lucky ones who will get early life-saving treatment.
- For more information about the Quest test, see the Useful addresses section at the end of the book.

JANE'S STORY
Six years ago, Jane, 47, discovered she had cancer of the cervix.

'I always attended for regular smears every three years, and these had always been clear. But I was about a year off from my next smear when I started to bleed between periods. I also felt very tired and generally unwell. I don't like going to my doctor, so instead I booked myself an appointment at a Well Woman clinic.

'The smear test they did was returned with borderline changes and I was told to have another smear in six months' time.

'I stopped worrying then. . . . But, the following month, I had the same old heavy period, spotting, headaches and lethargy. So this time I went to my GP. I was told the result would take six weeks to come through and this worried me a great deal. A lot of people might say I was over-reacting, but I decided to see a private doctor for a third opinion.

'The result of his smear was that I had cell changes and needed a colposcopy examination to see what was wrong.

'Within a few days, my GP's smear result came through with a completely different result: that I was all clear! I persuaded him, in the light of the private doctor's comments, to refer me to a gynaecologist and, luckily, a new consultant had just joined our local hospital and didn't have a long list so I saw him the following week.

'That's when I discovered I actually had a full-blown tumour –

and within ten days I was admitted for a hysterectomy.

'The interesting fact about all this is that three smears all taken around the same time came back with conflicting results. If I'd only had the GP's smear, I might have gone away thinking I was fine when, in fact, I was anything but. My consultant said that, six months on, my cancer might have spread to my lymph glands – in which case I might not have been here to tell the tale today.

'What I stress to anyone reading this is that, no matter what your result says, you should listen to what your body is telling you. I was bleeding and feeling unwell. If you are worried about your smear, seek a second opinion – or even a third one.'

2

Getting the results

After your smear test you will probably have to wait three to six weeks for the results to reach you, though, occasionally, they are returned much sooner. Your health authority may send you the results directly. Or, your doctor may telephone you with them. Some practices tell patients that they will not be contacted if the cervix has been found to be healthy. For your own peace of mind, you can always ring to check that the result was OK. And if you have waited more than six weeks for the results and are concerned, do chase them up. Several smear scandals in the last few years have meant women have assumed their result was normal, when, in fact, it never left the laboratory.

The result of your smear will tell you whether your result was normal or abnormal. It won't go into detail about abnormalities, but will suggest you see your doctor or that you arrange for a repeat smear.

If your result is normal, you have nothing to worry about and, providing your intuition is not telling you to pursue the matter further and you know you have no abnormal symptoms like bleeding or spotting or malaise (in which case see your GP or seek a second opinion from another source), you can forget all about smears until the next one is due.

If your result is abnormal, or positive, you will be invited to see your GP straight away for a chat.

This can be alarming, but is not always as sinister as it sounds.

The doctor has all the information about your smear result at his or her fingertips and should, in theory, be able to answer any of your questions about it.

Some doctors take the view that ignorance is bliss and that too much knowledge is frightening. Most women I have spoken to disagree with this. We are more frightened by what we *don't* know than what we *do*. We want to know what to expect – even the worst scenario.

Ask your doctor the following questions.

- What was found on the smear?
- What does this mean?
- Is any treatment necessary?
- What will that treatment be?
- Does it have any side-effects?
- Does it hurt?
- What is its success rate?
- What further treatment will I need if it fails?

Our minds race ahead – we want to feel prepared for what might happen to us in the future.

The doctor should be able to give you the following information about your smear.

- Whether or not the smear collected insufficient cells for analysis – a common reason for recall.
- Whether or not any infections, viruses, or other cervical abnormalities showed up on the smear. Infections such as thrush, gardnerella, trichomoniasis, and chlamydia, can all be reasons for recall after a smear – and all are easily treatable.

Thrush (or candidiasis) is a fungal infection that can cause a thick, white 'cottage cheese' discharge from the vagina, and vaginal itching and irritation. Antifungal creams or pessaries may be prescribed to treat it, and there are also many natural alternatives that are just as good.

Gardnerella is a bacterial infection of the vagina, which can be caused by stress or a change of sexual partner. The bacteria often causes an offensive, fishy smelling vaginal discharge, but clears up easily with the use of antibiotics.

Trichomoniasis is caused by an organism that can inhabit the vagina for years without causing symptoms. If symptoms do occur, they may include a yellow, frothy discharge and painful inflammation of the vagina and vulva. Treatment is with the antibiotic metronidazole and your doctor will probably ask to examine and treat your sexual partner at the same time to prevent reinfection.

Chlamydia is a very common sexually transmitted disease, which is often symptomless. It can be treated with antibiotics such as tetracyclines and erythromycin.

Viruses, such as the viruses that carry herpes and warts, are the most likely reasons for virus-related recall after a smear.

Herpes is a sexually transmitted disease that produces a painful rash on the genitals, itching, burning, soreness – and tiny blisters that burst and leave small ulcers. These heal in two to three weeks after an attack. But, having entered the body, the virus stays there for the rest of the sufferer's life – even though about 12 to 20 per cent of affected people never have another attack after the first. Even if you have several attacks in your first few years with the virus, these will gradually become less severe. Antiviral drugs encourage the ulcers to heal less painfully and bathing the area with salt water can help to reduce inflammation. If you are diagnosed as having herpes, your doctor should recommend that you have cervical smears annually.

Warts are growths that can appear anywhere on the body. They are caused by the human papilloma virus (HPV). There are over 75 strains of HPV. Some create warts on the cervix and a few are particularly fast-moving. A link between HPV and cervical cancer is known to exist and it is therefore important to receive treatment if it is recommended, or to attend for regular smears to check on the progress of your condition if that is what your doctor suggests.

- Whether or not there is any erosion (cervical ectropian) of the cervix. The cells on the surface of the cervix are hard, while those on the inside are softer. If these soft cells come to the surface (as can happen during ovulation, pregnancy or during a period) and if you have symptoms such as a discharge or bleeding between periods, you may need the condition treated. The treatment is the same as treatment for pre-cancerous cell changes to the cervix, which are discussed in Chapter 4.

- Whether or not any pre-cancerous cell changes were detected, and, if so, what stage these were found to be.

  Pre-cancerous cell changes are known as CIN (short for cervical intraepithelial neoplasia) or dysplasia (also known as dyskaryosis). Your GP will have been told by the laboratory whether this was CIN 1, CIN 2, or CIN 3. This scale shows the extent to which the cervix is affected.

  CIN 1 is mild dysplasia and indicates that a few cells in your smear showed changes. This condition may need treatment, or it may clear up on its own.

  CIN 2 is moderate dysplasia and would indicate that more than half the cells in your smear showed changes. Your doctor will probably refer you for a colposcopy examination.

  CIN 3 is severe dysplasia and shows that more than half the cells in your smear test had altered. Your doctor will definitely refer you for a colposcopy.

- Carcinoma *in situ* means that the changes found are quite extensive but have not yet 'invaded' and are therefore not 'cancerous'. At this stage you can be treated easily, but it is essential that you receive treatment now to avoid more serious problems. Carcinoma *in situ* means that the abnormal cells are still safely confined to the surface skin of the cervix. If you liken this stage to a ripe fruit that is about to burst, you can see how important it is to get treatment before the abnormal cells have a chance to spill out and 'invade' surrounding tissue.

- Invasive carcinoma means that the abnormal cells have spread beyond the surface of the cervix and the treatment you receive may be more involved than at the pre-cancerous stages. We will look at the possibilities for treatment at this stage in Chapter 4.

Even knowing, as you do now, that the majority of conditions detected on your smear test and for which you may be invited for a repeat smear or a chat with your GP are not life-threatening, you will be understandably alarmed if your result comes back with anything other than a 'Clear', 'Negative' or 'Normal' result.

Most of us only have to see the words 'abnormal', 'call your GP' or 'repeat smear' and we can see ourselves dead and buried!

This is particularly so when we receive a two-line letter from our

GP or health authority informing us the smear result was abnormal and should be repeated in six months' time.

I remember receiving a note to this effect from my health authority several years ago on a Saturday morning. It informed me that the smear I'd had a month earlier had a slightly abnormal result and that I might like to talk to my doctor about it.

As it was the weekend, I couldn't make an immediate appointment and went into a complete state of panic. I was convinced I was going to die, and was not at all reassured by my mother and sister, who both laughed at my anxiety when I phoned them. They pointed out that abnormal changes often return to normal and that the worst that could happen was I'd be referred to a specialist for treatment to remove the abnormal cells. My sister, who is six years younger than me, had already had this treatment and assured me there was nothing to it. But I remained unconvinced. I booked myself the earliest appointment I could get with my GP, and felt quite silly when he explained that my result hadn't even registered on the scale of pre-cancerous changes. It was simply that the cells had been difficult for the laboratory to analyse – probably because of the presence of mild thrush, which I hadn't even been aware of.

I had a repeat smear, the result was fine, and that was the end of that.

Now, having talked to women about their experiences for this book, I know that I am not alone in having got myself into such a state.

Far happier are the women whose GPs kindly intercept the results and make the effort to call them in person.

Of course, it can still be alarming to get a call out of the blue from your GP. But, handled the right way, he or she is the best person to put you at your ease at this distressing time.

DIANA'S STORY
Diana is 36 and has four children. Just after the birth of her youngest son, five years ago, she had a routine cervical smear.

'I've been with the same GP for years, and have always got on very well with him. When my result came through, he phoned me in person. His voice was calm and reassuring, but he said, "Now I've received your result, Diana, and it's not too good. It's CIN 3, which can be pretty serious if it's left untreated. But we've found it now, and the best thing is to get it treated as soon as possible. I'm making an appointment for you with a gynaecologist for laser treatment . . ."

'I know now that CIN 3 is the last stage of pre-cancer. But my doctor was so calm about the whole thing, I didn't get myself in a panic at all. I had the laser treatment, and now go for once-a-year smears. And so far they have all been perfectly normal.'

Diana's GP was wonderful, and many other doctors could take a leaf out of his book of bedside manners. But it is often not until we are faced with a bad news situation that we discover that our GP, who has dealt well with our sore throats and babies' injections for years, is not the reassuring person we thought he or she was.

TRACEY'S STORY
Tracey is a 27-year-old mother with two children.

'Where I live, smears are only offered once every five years. In the past I have asked for them to be carried out more regularly, but the answer has always been that I am not entitled to more frequent smears.

'My five years were up just after the birth of my son two years ago and I booked an appointment for a smear with my practice nurse.

'She said my cervix looked healthy and there should be no problems. But I was naturally quite worried when, nine-and-a-half weeks later, the result still hadn't come through. I phoned my doctor, desperate to know if I was clear or not, because I had a gut feeling it wouldn't be, and the receptionist said, "Ah, yes. . . . It is abnormal. Can you pop in and see the doctor?"

'By the time I saw him, I was in turmoil. He said I had CIN 3, the nucleus of the cell had changed and in his opinion it was the first stage of confined cancer.

'I was absolutely numb with shock. At my age, and having just had my second child, I'd thought I had my whole life ahead of me. Now I felt it was being snatched away from me and there was nothing I could do about it.

'I had tears in my eyes and the doctor was not at all comforting. He said, "You can talk to the receptionist about it if you like." I couldn't imagine why on earth he'd suggested that, but, much later, I discovered she had breast cancer and he thought the two of us would have something in common!

'Then he said I was to call him if I hadn't heard from the hospital within four weeks – and if I didn't get treated immediately I'd have full-blown cancer in six to twelve months and could be dead by the age of 35.

'I left the surgery in a daze. I was convinced I was doing to die. I'm 5 foot 10 inches tall and normally weigh over 9 stone, but I was so worried I couldn't eat a thing and my weight dropped to 7 stone. I couldn't look at my baby or touch him. I couldn't play with my five year old. I was a complete wreck.

'My husband wanted to take me out and buy me clothes. But I thought, what's the point if I'm going to die?

'In fact, I did make friends with the doctor's receptionist, and she helped me get a quick appointment with the gynaecologist. I don't know how I would have coped without her.

'I had laser treatment, and I am better now. But I still feel very angry with my GP. If he'd been more positive I would also have been more optimistic. Every day I think about the other women, like me, who have to go and see him to discover they have an abnormal smear result, and I feel so sorry that they are about to receive the same off-hand and off-putting treatment. But what can I do? Somebody warned me that if I made a complaint about the way he handled me, I'd risk being struck off his list. But someone's got to tell him how to talk to his patients!'

Getting the best out of your GP

- Prepare yourself with a list of questions about your smear.
- Don't worry about appearing ignorant or about asking silly questions. Your GP will respect you for asking and may only be used to giving information when asked for it.
- If you are worried about the news you are about to receive, ask if your partner, mother or friend can attend the consultation with you. They will be able to ask questions you may be too shocked to pose.

They will also take in information that you forget, and will later be able to discuss with you aspects of the consultation you may have misunderstood.

- Ask your GP if he or she knows of any support groups for counselling, if you think this would help, or if there is any further information to help you cope with the result or follow-up treatment. A lot of women complain that groups and information exist for people with cancer, but not for those with pre-cancerous changes. To discover you have these changes can be as traumatic as learning that your condition is more serious, so it is normal to need some kind of support. The experiences shared in this book will show you that you are not alone in feeling the way you do. At the end of the book, the Useful addresses section will help you find the support you need. If your GP is unable to offer this advice, show him or her this book and the lists at the back. You may be able to help the next woman who walks into that surgery after a positive smear.

VIVIENNE'S STORY
Vivienne is 36 and had a borderline smear result.

'In my area we have to call our GP's receptionist for smear results. When I did this six months ago, she came back to the phone groaning that it was "borderline".

'I was horrified. "What does that mean?", I asked. "Oh nothing really," she said. "Millions come back like this. But if you're worried you can come and see the nurse to talk about it."

'I didn't hang around, I got straight down there and the nurse reassured me that it was absolutely nothing to worry about and would probably go back to normal within six months. But I am a born worrier and I couldn't stop myself from agonizing about it.

'In the end, my husband convinced me to go to the doctor about it. She's a lovely lady doctor, and we knew she'd answer any questions we had.

'We sat down together and made a list, and Steve came with me.

'The doctor's exact words were, "This is so trivial that it's not worth the brain power to worry about it. It's probably just an infection you weren't even aware of."

'I actually came away feeling like a complete prune for having got myself in such a twist about nothing. But she didn't make me feel I'd wasted her time. And because Steve and I had already worked out our questions, she took us seriously and did her best to put us at our ease.'

3

What next?

Unless your GP has diagnosed an infection that needs immediate treatment, one of two things will happen to you now: either you will be asked to return for a repeat smear in six months' time or you will be referred to a colposcopy clinic.

Six months may seem a long time to wait when you are already very worried about your recent result. The reason you are asked to wait this long is that your cell changes are borderline, or CIN 1, and are expected to return to normal. Six months will give them time to do this, and the doctor will then check again that they are either back to normal or that no further deterioration has taken place.

If you are unhappy about waiting so long or at this point, like Jane in Chapter 1, want a second opinion, by all means ask for one.

Your options now

- A smear at a charitable status centre, like the British Pregnancy Advisory Service (see Useful addresses).
- A free smear in a Women's Nationwide Cancer Control Campaign mobile screening unit, if one happens to be in your area or at your workplace.
- A private smear or colposcopy.

Marie Stopes and some other clinics also offer something called cervicography. This is a technique in which a photograph is taken of the cervix, which has already been painted with a solution of acetic acid. The photographs are projected on to a screen and magnified so that the practitioner can see any abnormalities straight away. Some abnormalities that have not shown up in smear tests have been detected via cervicography. Cervicography is carried out in conjunction with colposcopy, so it shouldn't be necessary to have two separate investigations.

Whether you decide to postpone or speed up treatment, or if you are referred immediately, your mind is bound to find time to start dwelling on questions about the cause of your condition. I will discuss the possible causes of pre-cancer and cancer in more detail in Chapter 7, but it is worth passing on here the advice given by Queen's Medical Centre at Nottingham University Hospital, which is that women are more vulnerable to these conditions if:

- they do not have regular smears, every three years;
- they smoke – smoking reduces the number of barrier cells that defend your body against disease, and increases your risk of developing abnormal cells;
- they are infected with the human papilloma virus (HPV), or wart virus, which is sexually transmitted and has been linked with the development of CIN cells;
- their diet is unhealthy.

Having a colposcopy

A colposcopy will be recommended if there is any abnormality in your smear. It takes about five to ten minutes and is similar to a smear test, except that the doctor gets a much closer look at the cervix through a colposcope, which has a miscroscope lens.

LINDA'S STORY
Linda was referred for a colposcopy after an abnormal reading on her cervical smear test.

'I've never been happy about the current five-year rule for cervical smear tests, and when my GP gave me a postnatal smear test after the birth of my second daughter, Michelle, I asked him if he really believed it was all right to wait so long before next being screened.

' "Of course it is!", he said, then added, "Though you always get a few neurotic women who think they should be tested more often."

'His message to me was loud and clear – if I wanted a more regular check-up, I should go elsewhere for it. So, when, three years later, I decided to have another smear, I took myself to the local Well Woman clinic.

'I thought little more about the test . . . until my GP phoned me with news that the clinic had sent him my results and they were not good. He asked me to go in and see him, which I did, and I think he was almost as shocked as I was by the result. In such a short time, my smear reading had gone from normal to CIN 3, the most severe of the pre-cancer abnormalities. I dreaded to think what would have happened if I had waited another two years, but was relieved that treatment was at least available to me before invasive cancer had been allowed to develop.

'The doctor said the first step was to refer me to the colposcopy clinic, where (using a colposcope, which is a binocular microscope) a specialist could get a better look at the abnormal cells and then decide on treatment.

'I only had to wait a few weeks for the appointment to come through, but it felt like an eternity. Every time I switched on the television I seemed to hear about young mothers who had died from cancer, and half of me imagined this was to be my fate, while the other half was tempted to believe it was all some ridiculous mistake. I felt perfectly well, after all, so maybe the clinic had sent my GP somebody else's results.

'But when the day of my colposcopy finally came, it was clear there was no mistake at all.

'I had read everything I could on the subject of cervical cancer, so I knew what to expect – a glorified smear, really. I also fired questions at the doctor, which I'm sure would have remained unanswered if I had not bothered.

'The doctor looked down the colposcope at my cervix, then did a "punch biopsy", taking samples of the tissue from different points. Some women don't feel this at all, but I found it quite uncomfortable. The good thing was, the procedure only took a few minutes, and I also felt that I was in the best possible hands and that everything abnormal would be identified and dealt with as necessary.

'Despite the fact that I'd had a CIN 3 result, for which some women have to be hospitalized for a cone biopsy or diathermy, I was referred for out-patient treatment using laser therapy, which – less painfully than the punch biopsy – removed all the abnormal cells.

'A few weeks later I discovered that a colleague at work had had a similar smear result, though her treatment was more complicated. We decided to set up a helpline for other women facing colposcopies as a result of an abnormal smear. They are always very frightened when they first call. The best thing I can tell them is that my treatment took place over six years ago, and I have had no recurrence of abnormal cells since then.'

What is it?

A colposcopy is a magnified inspection of the cervix and vagina, used to identify or exclude the presence of pre-cancerous cells or early cancer in the cervix after an abnormal CIN result from a smear test.

How is it done?

You will probably be asked to put your legs in leg rests, while the doctor uses a speculum to hold the vaginal walls apart for the examination. A light is then shone down the passage on to the cervix. After taking a smear test, the doctor will dab the cervix with different liquids, which will show up the features of the cells. None of this is likely to hurt, though you may be a bit uncomfortable and feel some stinging. The doctor (or colposcopist) will then take several examples of surface tissue to send for examination in the path lab, as a further check.

A photograph may also be taken as a record. The examination takes about ten minutes. The doctor or colposcopist can normally reassure you straight away if there is no cancer present. If abnormal cells are confirmed, he or she can use a diagram to show you where they are and recommend treatment.

You may have very light bleeding for 24 to 48 hours after your colposcopy. During this bleed you should use a towel instead of tampons. You should also not have sex until the bleeding has stopped. This will allow the cervix to heal.

Colposcopic examination during pregnancy

Although you should ideally have a smear test *before* becoming pregnant, smears and colposcopic examinations during pregnancy are safe and will identify or rule out any abnormalities or cancer.

Pregnancy is not thought to affect the progress of CIN, but it can accelerate the progression of an invasive cancer (see Donna's story, page 59).

A biopsy is usually avoided during pregnancy because of bleeding, but if invasive cancer is suspected, a biopsy may be used to enable the appropriate management decisions to be made.

4

If you need pre-cancer treatment

Your colposcopy investigation should have been painless. Usually the only pain felt is if a punch biopsy sample of tissue is taken, and the colposcopist will have done this if abnormal cells have shown up during the examination. The solution applied to the cervix for the investigation causes pre-cancerous cells to show up white or with a surface pattern against the pink of normal healthy cells.

If the biopsy sample shows abnormal growth, you will require treatment.

The treatments

If the whole of the abnormal tissue can be seen during colposcopy, the abnormal tissue can be destroyed by laser, diathermy, or (although less common these days) cryosurgery.

A cone biopsy is a more far-reaching treatment, and tends to be used if the abnormal area is within the cervical canal and out of the sight of the colposcope.

- *Loop diathermy* removes the abnormal cells without destroying them so that a sample can be sent to the laboratory and examined under a microscope. The treatment only takes a few minutes and the doctor will use a local anaesthetic to numb the area. The loop usually only causes light discomfort, which may feel like a burning sensation, but this should only last a couple of seconds. Some women feel a pain similar to a period cramp during treatment – if this happens to you, your nurse will give you a painkiller.

- *Laser treatment* also takes only a few minutes and very efficiently removes the area of abnormal surface tissue on the cervix by focusing a very intense beam of light on it which vaporizes it. As it can be directed very accurately, it shouldn't disturb the rest of the cervix. The treated area takes a few weeks to heal, with new, healthy tissue growing over the area. To lessen the pain, a local anaesthetic is used before treatment starts. This is sometimes more painful than the treatment itself.

- *Cryosurgery* (or freezing treatment) is a slower and gentler treatment, but it is not as accurate or as efficient as laser. It takes about 10 to 15 minutes and may cause some flushing and aching, but this shouldn't last too long.

Take the day off work if possible so you can rest after the treatment. A period-like pain may be caused by the cervical canal contracting in response to the treatment on the cervix. You will probably also have a watery discharge for up to three weeks and will need to wear a sanitary towel. The discharge is the result of the surface tissues weeping, which they do when they are burned.

- *A cone biopsy* is used to remove the part of the cervix with the abnormal area of surface tissue (roughly in a cone shape 1.5 cm deep). The operation is minor, but can sometimes involve a hospital stay of up to three or even five days. After the operation, the vagina may be packed with wadding, which will be removed before you leave hospital. You may have stitches in your cervix (depending on the size of the incision) and these are usually dissolvable. If they are not, which would be unusual, they will be removed when you return to the hospital for a check-up.

After the operation, try to take some time off and take it easy for a couple of weeks. Bleeding is normal, but shouldn't become too heavy.

A disadvantage is that the cervix may not be quite so strong after a cone biopsy and, because of the risk of miscarriage, some women require a cervical stitch during a subsequent pregnancy.

Laser treatment

SARAH'S STORY

'My doctor only does smear tests on a five-yearly basis. After the last one, I received a note asking me to see him for the results.

'When I got there, he barely looked at me as he said, "I've booked you in for laser treatment tomorrow. You've got pre-cancerous cells". Then he looked at me and smiled and said, "Don't worry!" But I *was* worried! I was terrified!

'I went home feeling hysterical, but fortunately my sister knew someone who had had laser treatment. She told me all about it and, although I was still very nervous, at least I knew what to expect.

'The doctor who did my colposcopy was a young trainee and he wasn't at all reassuring. He seemed to be humming and hawing and said, "Mmm, it's quite bad!"

'I was horrified. "Do you think I'll need a hysterectomy?", I asked.

"That's something you'll have to discuss with the consultant," he said.

'Then the real consultant arrived, and he was lovely. His nurse was great, too. She kept me chatting all through the treatment, trying to take my mind off it. But it was difficult for me to let go, because I found the laser quite painful. I was very tensed up, which didn't help. And I could smell the burning, which was upsetting.

'When it was over, the nurse brought me a cup of tea and I was allowed to go home.

'A discharge is expected, but I actually started to haemorrhage the next day and had to go back into hospital. The consultant apologized and said this was very unusual. But I was so relieved to have the CIN 3 cells removed, I didn't care about anything else.

'I didn't attempt to have intercourse for at least three weeks after the treatment. And when I did, I found it very sore the first time.

'Everything's fine now, though. And I receive regular smears. So I really do feel I'm being well looked after.'

FIONA'S STORY

'I felt everything drain from me when my GP rang to say I'd had an abnormal smear. It was a total shock.

'She said she wanted to get things moving quickly so she was booking me in for a hospital appointment. Before I went in, she asked me to go and see her and she was able to answer all my questions about the treatment, and even drew me diagrams to show me what would happen. So by the time I got to hospital, I was well informed.

'The colposcopist said I would need laser treatment because there were some cells he couldn't see. My appointment came through a few weeks later and I was linked up to a TV screen so I could actually see the laser treatment in progress. My cervix started off looking like a cervix, and ended up like a barbecued beefburger, which was rather alarming.

'I got up feeling a bit shaky and was given a list of dos and don'ts to help my recovery and a prescription for iodine suppositories to use every night to aid healing.

'The healing process was, in fact, very rapid. By day three after treatment, all the "burned beefburger" tissue had been shed and I knew that new, healthy tissue was forming.'

Loop diathermy

WINIFRED'S STORY

'I've lived in England for five years. Before that I had spent my life in Scotland, where all women receive three-yearly smears. This was the first time I had to wait five years between checks and I was annoyed when I discovered that, from being normal, in five years my cells were CIN 2/3.

'It occurred to me that maybe my last smear had been a false negative. But, if five years ago I'd been told I had a positive smear, I might never have had my second baby. So, ultimately, I have no regrets about that.

'I was in a state of shock for about three days after getting the result, but my GP was very helpful. She drew diagrams of the cells and explained what had happened. Basically, on a scale of one to eight, I was at four.

'I decided to do more research of my own: if I've got to have a crisis, I like it to be a well-informed one!

'The doctor had told me I could have to wait three months for treatment. I soon discovered that some women wait even longer – up to six months. The doctor had also said that private treatment was costly. But, by ringing around, I discovered I could have a colposcopy and loop diathermy together for a total of £380. What's more I could be seen by a very good consultant within a fortnight.

'I'd read enough by now to know I wanted loop diathermy in preference over other treatments because I didn't like the idea of the tissue being destroyed, which is what happens when you have laser. If the tissue is removed with the loop, you can see the normal cells around it – and you know that they are OK and that there is nothing abnormal left.

'My treatment was done under local anaesthetic and it was no more uncomfortable than a visit to the dentist. I had that same feeling you have at the dentist of having loads of tubes in you, and a lot of prodding and poking going on as the doctor uses his speculum, probe and swabs. But it wasn't painful.

'The anaesthetic was also much the same as a dental anaesthetic. And, by way of proof that the whole procedure was painless, my husband, who was sitting in the next room, could hear me laughing and joking with the doctors.

'The doctors removed three layers of tissue. I asked to see them and it was like a tiny piece of layered tissue paper. It was very reassuring that this was all it was.

'I did heal up very well after the treatment, but I think that is because I took the doctor's advice very seriously. I took two weeks off work and relaxed on the sofa, reading and listening to the radio. I had a slight discharge for a fortnight, but nothing to worry about. You are more likely to start bleeding if you're on your feet a lot. I thought the new cells needed to be given time to establish themselves and I believe the rest I took helped that process.'

Cone Biopsy

JANE'S STORY
'I had a CIN 3 smear result 18 months after a clear one and, after being referred for a cone biopsy, I sat at home and worried myself sick.

'I should have taken this time to find out a bit more about what was going to happen. Instead, I went into hospital knowing something was going to be chopped off – and that was as far as it went.

'I was given a general anaesthetic and woke up two hours later still feeling too dazed to ask much about what the doctor had found.

'A month later, at my follow-up check-up, the consultant pronounced me fit and healthy and said I could go away and have annual smears.

'At the first of these, the nurse took one look at my cervix and said, "Yeuch!" – it was an unusual colour and eroded after the surgery. That worried me a lot. But it turned out to be fine, and quite normal after a cone biopsy.

'Since then, a lot of friends have called me for advice when they have needed treatment, and I also give talks about smears and treatment in schools.

'I am able to tell women that although I went into treatment ignorant of the details. I was quite well afterwards – not too sore and I recovered quickly. That always puts minds at rest.'

HELEN'S STORY

'When I was 25 years old, I decided to stop taking the Pill, and this seemed like a good time for a general overhaul. I asked my GP for a smear and I remember him saying I wasn't due one but he'd do it anyway.

'I never did get the result, and it didn't enter my mind to worry about it. But four or five months later, a note came from my GP asking me to pop in and see him about it. It turned out that the smear had been abnormal, and it was usual to repeat it after six months.

'This time the result came back with a CIN 2 reading and I was referred to a consultant. The upshot of all this was that, back then, laser treatment was still relatively new, and the consultant was a bit ambivalent about it and recommended a cone biopsy.

'It's not the most comfortable thing I've ever had done and I felt completely weak and useless following the general anaesthetic.

'My biggest worry, though, was my age and the severity of the treatment. A cone biopsy can weaken the cervix and make future pregnancies difficult. I didn't have any children at the time, but I guessed I would want them in the future and I didn't like to think my chances would be hindered. There is little or no way of knowing whether the muscle at the top of the cervix joining the uterus has been damaged until you try to have a baby.

'I was hugely worried, but, at a later colposcopy appointment, when I needed a cervical polyp removed, my consultant was reasonably confident that my muscle hadn't been damaged.

'At 34, I became pregnant and my husband and I worried even more about miscarriage. In the event, though, I had an easy pregnancy and worked until a fortnight before the baby was born – though I made sure everyone knew about my history, just in case a problem arose.'

After treatment

- Do not use tampons and avoid intercourse until the discharge has stopped.
- If you have a discharge, use a sanitary towel.
- If you bleed or have a very heavy discharge, see your doctor.
- Take a daily bath to help prevent infection.
- Eat a healthy diet with plenty of green vegetables, carrots and fresh fruit. This will promote the growth of healthy healing cells.

The biggest worry after treatment is that the cells, although now normal, may become pre-cancerous again. If something caused this to happen once, what's to stop it doing the same thing again?

The development of abnormal cells probably results from several factors coming together at one time, with something triggering off the unhealthy growth. The same combination of factors is unlikely to happen again. Even if it did, the body's defence mechanisms may be able to deal successfully with the condition without medical intervention. But regular smear tests will provide you with early warnings if any changes do occur and these will be treated before they can become harmful.

Cervical incompetence

What is the risk of treatment to your future fertility?

If the cervix is abnormally weak, following treatment, the weight of the fetus may cause the cervix to begin gradually to open around the twelfth week of pregnancy, when it should be staying closed until you go into labour. Cervical incompetence is normally suspected if a woman has had two or more miscarriages after the fourteenth week of pregnancy, and about one in five women who have recurrent miscarriages after 14 weeks have cervical incompetence. If an incompetent cervix is suspected, during the fourth month of pregnancy, you can have the cervix stitched closed. A stitch is tied around the cervix like a purse string, and the operation is done either under epidural or general anaesthetic. The stitch is left in place until the end of the pregnancy and then cut so that you can deliver the baby normally.

KAREN'S STORY

'I had my first baby – a bouncing boy – 7 years ago, when I was 30 years old. The pregnancy went like a dream. I was very healthy and active all the way through, and there were no complications with the birth. Everything was just as it should be: a textbook pregnancy.

'Harry was three years old when my smear was returned with abnormal results, and my consultant recommended a cone biopsy. I didn't know anything about this procedure at the time, except that, as he said, it was the most certain way to get rid of anything sinister lurking in my cervix, and that was good enough recommendation for me to go ahead with it.

'But, following the cone biopsy, I suffered two miscarriages – both pretty late in pregnancy. The first, at 22 weeks, and, horrendously, while I was on holiday in the Canaries. I lost the second baby at 20 weeks, a year later.

'Neither miscarriage pointed directly to a fault with the cervix, but, after reading up on the subject from a book I got from the Miscarriage Association, I started to think this might be the cause. So, when I was pregnant for the fourth time, I asked for a cervical stitch, and this was put in at 14 weeks, under general anaesthetic.

'The stitch was removed at 38 weeks and the consultant commented that William was born very rapidly after its removal, which makes me wonder how my cervix would have coped and if I would have suffered the trauma of a third miscarriage had the stitch not been in place.

'Not everyone needs a cervical stitch after a cone biopsy – and it is unlikely you would be offered one prior to having suffered at least one miscarriage – but it is good to know that this is something available to women whose cervixes have been weakened as a result of previous treatment. And I was certainly very pleased to think that something so simple saved my baby.'

5

What if it's cancer?

Before sitting down to write this chapter, I was watching a TV drama in which Nancy, a young mother, goes to her doctor to ask about going back on the Pill. While they chat, Nancy mentions a spot of lower back pain she's been having, which she thinks she has inherited from her father's side of her family. To be on the safe side, the doctor says she'll check it out. It turns out to be cancer, in Nancy's case ovarian cancer.

What Nancy goes through in this storyline mirrors very closely the experiences of women I have spoken to about cervical cancer. One day you are happily jogging along, never even imagining there can be anything wrong with you. The next, while undergoing a routine check-up, you learn you have a life-threatening malignancy. With this discovery, all sorts of thoughts go through your mind.

- 'Yesterday I was OK. Today I am not – if I hadn't come in for this routine check, I never would have known – and my life would still be as it was yesterday.'
- 'I haven't got time for this now – I'm too busy with my life to get cancer.'
- 'I'm young and healthy – I don't *feel* ill, and I can't believe I *am* ill. It's got to be a mistake.'
- 'Am I going to die?'

A MacMillan nurse who works closely with women who have cervical cancer told me that this form of cancer, more than any other, has an enormous psychological impact on women. There are often no symptoms, so it is hard for patients to believe that they are really ill. They are embarrassed about the location of the cancer, because of its sexual connotations. Their body image suffers a serious blow, which can destroy their self-confidence. And they are shocked at the nature of the surgery that will be involved in their treatment.

All this means they tend not to ask too many questions, and not to put up too much of a fight to get the kind of individual treatment that, say, a breast cancer patient may demand for herself. Only the minority of cervical cancer patients demand one treatment over another. Most willingly put themselves in the hospital's hands and go along with whatever their consultant deems appropriate.

However, there are options and decisions to be made and, in this chapter, I hope to explain these choices and to help you come to the right decision about your treatment.

First of all, though, let's look at the meaning of the term cancer of the cervix.

We have already seen that there are three main stages (CIN 1, 2 and 3) of pre-cancer of the cervix. What happens next is that CIN 3 or carcinoma *in situ*, left untreated, stands a 20 to 30 per cent chance of progressing to invasive cancer. This means that the cells which are cancerous have penetrated beyond the surfce of the cervix. In many cases, invasive cancer will produce symptoms such as pain. But it is possible to have invasive cancer without these symptoms – especially in the earlier stages of the disease. For, just as there are different stages of pre-cancer, invasive cancer progresses through different stages. The exact stage one patient's cancer has reached is determined by means of physical examinations, lymphograms, intravenous urograms, ultrasound, CAT scans and NMR.

The stages, classified by the International Federation of Obstetrics and Gynaecology are as follows:

- Stage 1a (microinvasive carcinoma) – the cancerous cells have broken through the basement membrane of the cervix, but are not yet widespread
- Stage 1b – the cancerous cells have broken through to beyond 5mm from the basement membrane and the lymphatic channels may be involved
- Stage 2a – the cancer has spread into part of the vagina
- Stage 2b – the cancer has spread into tissue around the cervix
- Stage 3 – the lower vagina and pelvic wall are also involved
- Stage 4 – the cancer has spread beyond the genital area and into nearby organs.

By 'staging' the cancer, the oncologist or surgeon can tell how

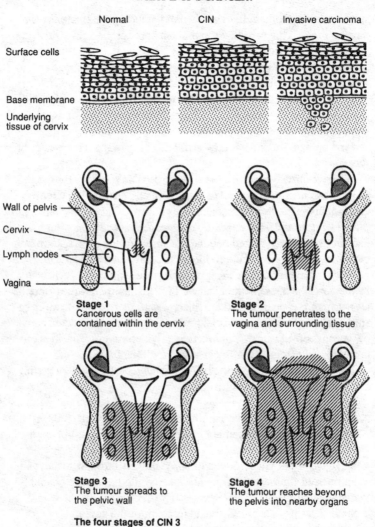

Normal   CIN   Invasive carcinoma

Surface cells

Base membrane

Underlying tissue of cervix

Wall of pelvis

Cervix

Lymph nodes

Vagina

Stage 1
Cancerous cells are contained within the cervix

Stage 2
The tumour penetrates to the vagina and surrounding tissue

Stage 3
The tumour spreads to the pelvic wall

Stage 4
The tumour reaches beyond the pelvis into nearby organs

The four stages of CIN 3

widespread the disease is, and how much tissue should be removed. This is vital because, if the extent of the cancer is underestimated, insufficient tissue may be removed and the cancer will continue to spread.

- A physical examination under anaesthetic allows the doctor to stage the cervical cancer, view the tumour, and take biopsies. He or she will also look into the bladder and rectum examining the bladder using a cystoscopy (viewing instrument) and the rectum using a protoscopy. Sometimes a D & C (dilatation and curettage) is performed. This means that a little of the lining of the uterus is scraped out for examination.
- In some units, a lymphogram is performed. This is a technique in which the abdomen and pelvis are X-rayed in order to identify lymph nodes in which tumour cells have lodged. Before the X-ray, radio-opaque dye is injected into the lymph channels in the feet and it then spreads around the body, outlining the lymph glands and highlighting tumours that would not normally be visible.
- An intravenous urogram (IVU) also involves radio-opaque dye – this time injected into a vein in the arm. It becomes concentrated in the urinary system and, under X-ray, highlights any blockage of the ureters – the tubes connecting the kidneys to the bladder.
- A computerized axial tomography (CAT) scan takes X-ray pictures from different angles so that a computer can build up a two-dimensional image of the body. This time, you will have to drink the radio-opaque liquid. It shows up any abnormalities on the X-ray. Also a tampon will be used to open the vagina slightly before the scan and often an intravenous injection will be given.
- A nuclear magnetic resonance (NMR) scan may also be offered. Strong magnetic waves are passed through the body and highlight tumours by causing a different reaction in them to the reaction of normal tissue. The differences show up on a computer-generated television image. The main problem with both NMR and CAT scans is that they are unable to detect tumours less than 1 cm in diameter.
- An ultrasound scan also picks up and shows images of abnormalities on a computer screen, but is not as accurate as a CAT or NMR scan.

Reacting to the news – personal experiences

VAL'S STORY

For Val, 46, everything happened so quickly she hardly had time to take it in.

'I've always been very aware of the need to have regular cervical smear tests and was due to have a smear when I began to bleed between periods.

'It was heavy enough to need sanitary protection, but not as heavy as a normal period. And, although I found it odd, because I'd never suffered anything like this before, I must admit I wasn't unduly worried. My mother had had her menopause in her early forties, and, at 44, I thought this must be the beginning of my own change.

'It was my sister who said I ought to have it checked out. I'd been having this mid-monthly bleeding for four months in a row when I mentioned it to her. And she said it sounded a bit funny and, even if it *was* hormonal, there would be no harm in talking to my doctor about it.

'Well, my doctor examined me straight away – and her first words were, "It doesn't look too good, Val."

'I think she probably suspected then that I had cancer, but she decided to take a smear anyway.

'Fortunately she is the kind of doctor who doesn't like to hang around and she also referred me directly to a consultant gynaecologist at our local hospital. Because, if I'd waited for the result of the smear to come through, I could easily have believed nothing was wrong with me!

'The result, when it arrived several weeks later, was "normal". . . . But, by this time I had undergone a hysterectomy!

'This isn't to say, of course, that *all* smears are unreliable. A lot of women's cancers are identified from their smear test. But in my case none of the cancerous cells appeared on the smear.

'I saw the consultant the day after my first appointment with my GP. She examined me and then asked me to come in for a biopsy so she could see what was going on.

'Looking back, the word "biopsy" should have rung warning

bells with me. . . . But, at the time, I still didn't put two and two together. I just went into hospital, as requested. And the biopsy was carried out under general anaesthetic.

'By the time the consultant came round with the results, I'd got to know all the nurses on the ward. We were all having a chat when she approached, looking grim, and said, "It's not good news", and they all fell silent. I looked at their faces, then at the consultant, and I burst into tears.

'I seem to have blocked out the rest of the conversation. I know I felt numb with shock at the time. But she explained that she had found a tumour – and that I would need a CAT scan and "staging" investigation to check that it hadn't spread any further than the cervix.

'The scanning machine at Newham General Hospital, where I was a patient, wasn't working. So I was transferred to the Royal Marsden.

'My cancer was an adenocarcinoma, which is the rarer type of cervical cancer – affecting only 10 per cent of women. And the good news, after all the bad news, was that the tumour was at stage 1b, which meant it was completely contained within the cervix. I remember the doctor coming to explain it to me. I was watching his hands as he spoke and he seemed to be indicating that it was about an inch big.

'He said that the best option for me was to have a hysterectomy because chemotherapy and radiotherapy would involve long-term treatment and sickness. But, if I didn't want surgery, the rate of cure was the same with radiotherapy.

'In fact, in any case where radiotherapy is a possibility, the cervix can be marked for treatment with four gold grains, and these had already been put in place.

'But I decided the hysterectomy was the better option.

'The operation was awful – I woke up feeling grottier than I've ever felt in my life, and for four days, the hospital staff commented on how lovely it was to have such peace on the ward because I was so quiet!

'But I had no regrets. None whatsoever. I felt satisfied I'd done the right thing. . . . Although I admit I was very frightened when I went for my first three-month check-up after the operation.

'Everything's fine now. I'm on to once-a-year checks. And my fear of cancer has subsided.

'It's funny, because, before my cancer, it had never occurred to me that I might get it. . . . Then, when I did, everything seemed to happen so quickly – I had three procedures (the biopsy, the CAT scan, and the hysterectomy) in less than a month – that I barely had time to think about what had hit me!'

REBECCA'S STORY
For Rebecca, 27, the news that she had cancer came as a bolt from the blue.

'I was 25 years old when I discovered I had cancer of the cervix – but I think I'd actually had it for some time when it was finally diagnosed.

'My very first smear was taken when I was 17 and pregnant with my eldest daughter. The result showed I had an eroded cervix with a "rather infected appearance" and "slight changes". A repeat smear after my baby was born showed there was still some inflammation, and I was asked to come back in a year's time. The result, a year on, was no different. But my doctor didn't seem too bothered by it.

'A year later, my second daughter was born, and the midwife made a note that she had spotted a small round nodule on my cervix. But she didn't mention this to me, and I only found out about it after my cancer was diagnosed, when I began to look into my history.

'I had one more inflammatory smear, and then, in November 1989, a negative result – at which point I was asked to come back in five years' time.

'In the light of what happened next, I find this absolutely horrifying.

'In February 1993, seven months into my third pregnancy, I suddenly started bleeding after intercourse.

'My GP didn't think it serious. But the second time it happened, I was so scared I decided to avoid intercourse for the rest of my pregnancy.

'A month later, I was doing housework when I suddenly began

to bleed, for no apparent reason. My husband drove me up to the hospital and I was examined by the gynae registrar who said he could feel something like a baby's foot on my cervix.

'My first thought was that the baby had suddenly moved into a breach position. But then the registrar went on to say, "But it's not a foot. . .".

'By this time all sorts of warning bells were ringing in my head. The consultant was called and he decided to induce labour. The baby was due in two weeks' time anyway, so I wasn't putting her in any danger.

'When she was born, the doctor wrote the word "polyp" in my notes and followed it with a question mark.

'My baby and I went home from hospital, and I was still none the wiser about what was happening to me. But, two weeks later, on my first attempt at intercourse in weeks, I bled so profusely that it was all over the bed. It looked dreadful. But I wasn't in any pain at all, which seemed strange.

'The GP said it was to do with the trauma of the baby's birth. She said this seven times in all over the next few months when the bleeding occurred.

'It was several months later when she finally referred me to hospital, telling the gynaecologist that I had a possible cyst because I was bleeding easily.

'But, before my appointment came, I was rushed to casualty with such tremendous loss of blood that I needed a blood transfusion. I was taken to theatre for a biopsy, and the result was a "moderately differentiated squamous cell carcinoma: stage 1b".

'The tumour itself was an 8-cm mass – four times the size of my cervix, so how it had gone undetected for so long, I can't imagine!

'The consultant didn't tell me the result of the biopsy. He left that job to my poor husband – who didn't have a clue where to start, or what to say.

'When he finally spat it out, I couldn't believe it. I was young. I'd just had a baby. I couldn't absorb the fact that I now had cancer.

'I was convinced I was going to die, that my two older daughters would grow up without me, and my baby would have no memory of me. I felt sorry for my family and sorry for myself at the thought that I wouldn't live to see them do all the things we plan for our children. It was a nightmare.'

Thankfully Rebecca did not die. Her story is continued later in this chapter.

JANE'S STORY CONTINUED
In Chapter 1, Jane told us how she discovered she had cancer. Here she explains how her positive attitude to the disease helped her.

'Most people are completely phased by their fear of cancer. I was no exception. I had read all I could on the subject and still managed to convince myself I didn't have the symptoms when, clearly, I did. Even so, I was doing something about finding out for sure. Which is, of course, after three separate smears, how I finally found out the truth.

'It was actually quite advanced when the diagnosis was made. It had already spread to the lymph nodes – and these were removed with my hysterectomy.

'I realized I'd been under a lot of stress at the time of developing the cancer, and I felt sure that this had contributed in some way. So I looked into ways of mobilizing my body's own self-healing processes.

'I was very confident that my surgeon had removed everything, but when he suggested I had follow-up treatment at London's Royal Marsden cancer hospital, I was not at all keen on the idea. I had been brought up to appreciate alternative and complementary medicine, and I really wanted to take a chance at doing things my way before going back for radiotherapy or chemotherapy.

'Persuading the doctors to let me do this was actually very difficult. I found I was almost *forced* to have radiotherapy, and when I refused, I was pushed on to the chemotherapists. . . . All of them kept saying that without this follow-up treatment, there was a 50:50 chance of the cancer coming back. I said, "No, I might be one of the 50 per cent who *don't* get the cancer back!" That is what I call positive thinking! And I eventually found a consultant who was also very positive, sympathetic, and willing for me to use complementary medicine if that was what I wanted.

'I felt very strongly that I wanted to make life more pleasant for myself. And that is exactly what I set out to do.'

An increasing number of specialist cancer units now have a MacMillan nurse on hand to guide patients through the minefield of emotions they experience at this frightening time. If you are lucky enough to have such a nurse, she or he will be able to help you, your partner, and your family to cope and make informed decisions about your treatment and other aspects of your illness.

The treatment of choice

Your specialist may talk about his or her 'treatment of choice' for you. This is a little bit like the 'best advice' that financial institutions give you when they have looked into your personal circumstances and assessed your individuals needs: the decision is based not only on your particular requirements, but also the hospital's facilities, budgets, research and current philosophy. Just as you have every right to reject your bank's 'best advice' for your financial future, you are entitled to ask your consultant to respect your wishes in the treatment you receive. By doing this you will not necessarily be jeopardizing your chances of a decent cure. But it is important that your decision is an informed one, and it may mean that you have to transfer to another hospital to get the treatment you want.

Except in circumstances where the cancer is confined and can be easily removed by means of a cone biopsy, the treatment of choice for early cervical cancer at St Bartholomew's Hospital in London is a radical hysterectomy, and, in Chapter 6, I examine in detail the pros and cons of this operation. In some other hospitals, the treatment of choice is radiotherapy. In many cases, patients require both – surgery followed by radiotherapy. But, if it is a simple case of either one *or* the other, which would you choose?

As Val said in her story above, everything can happen so quickly that you hardly have time to consider what is going to happen to you, and, when all you want is to get rid of the cancer, you may quite willingly succumb to any treatment your consultant recommends. But, the treatment does have long-term effects and it is you who will have to live with them.

Radiotherapy

There are two forms of radiotherapy for cervical cancer.

- Internal radiotherapy – in which small tubes or packets containing radioactive metals, such as caesium or cobalt, are placed in the vagina so that the radiation gets a direct hit on the malignant tissue. Depending on the type of radiotherapy being used, it can be quite a lonely process as it involves being left alone for long periods.
- External radiotherapy – in which a beam of high-energy gamma X-rays is directed at tumours. This involves short treatments spread over a period of weeks. It isn't as lonely as internal radiotherapy as it only takes seconds and is a bit like lying on a sunbed – except that it can make you feel nauseous.

Essentially, radiotherapy works by burning the malignant tissue, using doses of radiation, similar to, but many times more powerful than, the rays used for X-rays. This will give you some idea of the possible side-effects on healthy tissue that also comes into contact with the radiation.

Side-effects

- Vaginal changes are a major side-effect – the vagina shortens and narrows as a result of radiotherapy. There is reduced elasticity of the vaginal walls, and less lubrication. Sexual intercourse can become very difficult after radiotherapy. Vaginal dilators, used on a regular basis, can help considerably, but they can be uncomfortable and it is best to start using them, with the long term in view, as soon as possible after treatment. Even though you may not feel ready for sex for quite a while yet, you must consider that, later on, you will be. The ideal time to start using the dilators is three to four weeks after completion of treatment, and as they now come in pretty toiletry bag packs and are not as hideous as some of the old dilators women used to be given, they can be seen, even when you are feeling far from sexy, as an attractive option.

  The dilator is a plastic tube-like instrument, which comes in a variety of lengths and widths. The object of it is to keep the vaginal passage open, and most patients who use dilators will use them once a day. With the help of a lubricating jelly, you insert the dilator into the vagina and then move it about as much as you can for about two minutes.

HRT will also be prescribed after radiotherapy (see page 57).

- The bowel can also suffer – you may experience chronic diarrhoea, flatulence and colitis, or severe symptoms of irritable bowel syndrome. In a small number of cases, when the bowel and vaginal walls become fused after treatment (a fistula), a colostomy may become necessary, but this is rare (occurring in fewer than 1.2 per cent of cases).
- The bladder and urinary tract frequently suffer complications – cystitis is a common problem after radiotherapy, for example.
- Weight loss, nausea and anorexia are also seen in patients who have undergone radiotherapy.

Combined with the psychological fall-out of having had cancer, these physical symptoms can make life miserable and uncomfortable for a woman who, prior to diagnosis, had been carefree and independent.

REBECCA'S STORY CONTINUED

'In my mind there was no question of a cure. I thought I was going to die, and that was that. I felt as if I was going to burst with the trauma, my sadness was so great. I wanted the tumour removed immediately. Yesterday wouldn't have been soon enough! Then the doctor told me they were going to do it in a week – and that felt like a year away.

'I didn't question him when he told me I'd be having caesium implant radiotherapy rather than a hysterectomy. He warned me there was a slight risk of bowel damage. But by that I had no idea he meant that some women end up with a colostomy bag. Besides, right then, I just wanted rid of the tumour. I wasn't in any mood to think about side-effects, and, whatever they turned out to be, at the time I just wanted my life back.

'I was lucky – the radiotherapy shrunk all 8 cm of my tumour completely, and there hasn't been any sign of recurrence.

'But, now, I do wish I'd been told more about the side-effects. The front wall of my rectum is now stuck to my cervix, and this has given me extreme symptoms of irritable bowel syndrome. I swing between being constipated and suffering diarrhoea. I have mucus in my stools, and a lot of blood. And, yes, I've been told I might one day have to have a colostomy.

'I also leak urine without warning. And sex is impossible. I am only 26. My husband is 29. It's terrible for him. I look like the same person. He still wants to make love to me. But he can't. Only a third of my vagina is OK. The rest is all closed up, hardened and ulcerated. We've attempted intercourse and it's ended in failure. I've got dilators, but they're so uncomfortable I don't like to use them. It's a big, big problem with my marriage, and I've seen other couples split up over the after-effects of radiotherapy. I just pray it won't happen to me.'

It doesn't have to be like this. For some people, radiotherapy is the only treatment on offer. So how can you make the most of the experience?

FIONA'S STORY
Fiona started her course of external radiotherapy in a positive frame of mind. Here she describes how she 'made friends with' the treatment.

'Funnily enough, it never even occurred to me that death was on the cards. I think I had a very positive attitude to my treatment, and even my oncologist said that was half the battle.

'My radiotherapy hardly set me back at all. I even managed to continue working full time through it. I had early morning appointments, each one lasting under an hour. Then I would go straight off to work from the hospital.

'I even found the radiotherapy machine very friendly. You are carefully positioned under its beam, and treatment lasts only a few minutes. The machine makes a soft beeping noise, which is quite comforting really. It certainly wasn't anything to be frightened by.

'I had already studied the visualization techniques used at the Bristol Cancer Centre. These involve using your mind to imagine that the cancer cells are being destroyed. And, during my radiotherapy, I imagined my tumour as a corn or a wart that was being whittled down by a constant trickle of corrosive ointment.

'I'll never forget the joy on my consultant's face when my

treatment was finally over and the tumour had gone completely. He and his colleague were dancing around the room. They couldn't believe it!

'After weeks of battling on and running around on full steam, I went home, got drunk and called all my friends to tell them the good news. I knew the worst was over. And I was confident that I would survive.'

Questions about the treatment of cancer

Q. How does the cancer spread?

A. In early cancer, the malignant cells multiply and gradually push out normal healthy cells in the cervix. If they are not stopped early enough, they will continue to advance, like an army, into the body's lymph channels – a network of channels that carry immune white cells all around the body. These immune cells have the job of fighting any infection, bacteria, virus or malignancy that enters the body. But the lymph channels can also be used by the cancer cells to spread themselves around the body. They become trapped in lymph nodes and these can become swollen and tender. (However, normal infections are a much more common cause of swollen lymph nodes, so don't panic just because you find one slightly enlarged.) By using the lymph channels, the cancer cells travel to other sites in the body – and the more they spread, the harder it is to get rid of them.

Q. Can I have a baby after cancer treatment?

A. In the majority of cases, the straight answer to this question is 'no'. Radiotherapy makes conception impossible, and, in most cases, the only alternative to radiotherapy is a hysterectomy.

However, women in France are offered the chance to have only the cervix removed, and in a small group of women with very early disease this may become a future option for British women suffering early invasive cervical cancer. The removal of the cervix doesn't hinder a woman's chances to conceive in the normal way, and obviously has many bonuses for women who are still keen to start a family.

Q. When and why does chemotherapy become necessary?

A. Chemotherapy – the use of chemicals to kill the cancer cells – may be introduced if the cancer has spread into the lymph channels, but, while it has proved very effective for the treatment of many other cancers, it has not so far proved popular or particularly successful in the treatment of cervical cancer. New techniques that will single out cancer cells and target them for treatment may one day get rid of the need for radiotherapy and surgery, but it is more likely they will be used alongside these existing treatments.

Q. How successful is treatment likely to be?

A. If the cancer is caught *before* the lymph nodes are involved, there's an 80 to 90 per cent chance of cure. If the lymph nodes *are* involved, however, and the cancer has spread to other parts of the body, the chance of a cure is only 50 per cent, and half the women with later-stage cancers die within five years. So, it is important to detect changes early.

6

Hysterectomy

Although it can be very traumatic to lose a breast, in that it can be seen, it can seem just as bad to lose your internal organs, and to have the knowledge that there is nothing left of your secret womanhood. Jane Metcalf, *The Bristol Experience*

A hysterectomy may seem drastic but it can have advantages over radiotherapy.

Radiotherapy may be given as an out-patient and survival rates are similar to rates of survival after surgery. But, the psychological effect of having had the tumour removed through surgery is a bonus to many women: that malignant area has gone and, unless you are very unlucky, it will not return. There is also the fact that younger women can keep their ovaries, staging of the cancer is extremely accurate when surgery is performed, and an active sex life is more likely to continue because the vagina, while shortened, remains more pliable than after radiotherapy.

Now let's look at the disadvantages of radiotherapy *and* surgery. Radiotherapy can cause:

- the vagina to become dry, rigid and lacking in sensation
- urinary tract complications, including cystitis, urinary frequency and a contracted blader
- bowel complications, including chronic diarrhoea and flatulence
- ovarian ablation (damage to the ovaries), causing an early menopause.

There is also the risk of secondary cancer.

Hysterectomy can cause:

- the usual complications of a prolonged operation (mainly the risk of anaesthetic complications and haemorrhage)
- infection in the chest, wound, urinary tract and pelvis

- bladder and bowel problems
- sexual problems because of the now shortened vagina.

However, these problems are less likely to be long term or permanent than they would be after radiotherapy, but there is still the chance that you may need radio- or chemotherapy after surgery.

For most young women the main concern about having a hysterectomy is that they will no longer be able to have children. Sadly, both hysterectomy and radiotherapy for cervical cancer spell the end of one's childbearing years.

Having a hysterectomy

Cervical cancer is one medical reason for a woman having a hysterectomy. Others include endometriosis, pelvic inflammatory disease, fibroids and prolapse of the womb.

The type of hysterectomy operation performed will depend on the condition being treated.

A sub-total hysterectomy – in which only the womb is removed – is an operation rarely performed these days, mainly because it leaves the cervix as a potential site for cancer.

A total hysterectomy – often the choice of treatment for fibroids, endometriosis, prolapse or period problems – removes the cervix as well as the womb. The ovaries remain, which is important because they are responsible for producing the flow of monthly hormones, without which you would experience an early menopause. With the ovaries still intact, you will continue to produce progesterone and oestrogen in cycles as before. Having had your womb removed, you will not recognize this cycle in the way that you used to as you will no longer experience monthly periods, but the hormones play an important part in preventing the problems associated with menopause.

A total hysterectomy with bilateral salpingo-oophorectomy is given to women who have already passed the menopause and involves the removal of the ovaries and Fallopian tubes in addition to the uterus and cervix.

The radical or Wertheim's hysterectomy removes the cervix, the womb and the surrounding tissue, and the top of the vagina (then it is termed a radical hysterectomy) or the upper third of the vagina and the fatty tissue and lymph glands in the pelvis to which the cancer cells may have migrated (then called a Wertheim's hysterectomy). However, even with such extended surgery, it is sometimes possible – and desirable – to keep the ovaries, thus allowing normal hormonal cycles to continue.

For the treatment of cervical cancer, it is most likely that you will have this last type of hysterectomy.

How the operation is done

In some cases, especially if your hysterectomy is for a prolapsed uterus, the surgeon may approach the operation via the vagina. However, for the treatment of cervical cancer, where a radical or Wertheim's hysterectomy is required, the surgeon will want to open the abdomen to operate. This involves a horizontal or midline vertical cut.

In their natural state, the combined womb, ovaries and tubes are only the size of a pear and a couple of plums, and, once gone, the bladder and intestines move over and fill the space, so you are not left with a huge gap. The surgeon sews up the hole left by the removal of the cervix, so you need have no worries about your insides being open to infection. Everything is as well protected as before.

Women's feelings about hysterectomy

Before the operation

Even if you have had all the children you want, and even if you know that your hysterectomy is going to cure you of cancer, the prospect of surgery can be horrific. For one thing, the news that you have cancer is likely to have only just reached you, so you have a lot to take on board all at once. It is also a major operation, and it may seem to be getting in the way of your life because you have not had time to plan for it.

Also, as Suzie Hayman says in her book, *Hysterectomy*, 'the removal of your womb can seem to rip out the essence of your womanliness'.

After the operation

Everyone will warn you of the emotional fall-out you are likely to experience after hysterectomy. But many women find it hard to imagine how they will feel and, in spite of the warnings, are totally unprepared for their turbulent emotions. First, major surgery of any kind is stressful and many women become quite tearful in the first few weeks after their operation. Their sadness is often unrelated to their feelings about losing their womb and their physical recovery from the operation, but that is not to say that they may also be in a great deal of pain at this time.

Being prepared can at least help you understand *why* you are depressed and that, to some extent, will help you through this difficult time. A lot of women feel that their depression is linked to the lack of information they've been given, so find out as much as you can about your operation prior to going in to hospital. But, however well equipped you are when you go into the operation, some depression and loss of self-esteem is normal afterwards (See Personal experiences of hysterectomy, page 59).

Getting back to normal, physically

- Don't expect an immediate recovery. That will lead to disappointment and frustration.
- Feeling tired, exhausted and emotionally low are a normal part of early recovery.
- Give yourself plenty of rest.
- Build up your exercise routine slowly – a five-minute daily walk will be fine to begin with.
- Make sure you eat regularly (see also my advice on healthy eating on page 81).
- Sit to do small jobs about the house.
- Avoid heavy work – carrying shopping, vacuuming, moving furniture and driving.
- Keep up the pelvic floor exercises that your nurse or doctor should have explained to you.

If you need HRT
(Hormone Replacement Therapy)

HRT is prescribed when the ovaries have been removed and the body is then deprived of its natural supply of hormones.

Without HRT, postmenopausal women (and those who reach menopause prematurely because their ovaries have been removed) are at greater risk of bad health in old age. Osteoporosis (brittle bones), heart attacks and strokes are all commoner problems in women over the age of 50. HRT reduces the likelihood of these and other symptoms.

Many women say they would rather put up with menopausal symptoms because they are not life-threatening. But their quality of life is greatly impaired by succumbing to the effects of the menopause. Not only do they become irritable and moody, they are also likely to go off sex, become forgetful and suffer aching joints, hot flushes and night sweats. And these symptoms can continue for many years.

When you have your ovaries, the hormones they produce – oestrogen and progesterone – greatly influence your health and even your personality.

Oestrogen is the sexy or up-beat hormone. It makes you feel good and keeps you full of pep. Your body normally makes this throughout the month. Progesterone is the downbeat, mumsy, hormone that prepares you for pregnancy, and, if you get pregnant, keeps the pregnancy going.

When your body stops producing these hormones, you begin to experience withdrawal symptoms. Your temperature control system goes haywire, causing hot flushes and sweats. You feel listless and tired and irritable with your family. And you start to feel the signs of ageing – aches and pains, sudden wrinkles, dry hair and even forgetfulness.

HRT treats these symptoms by 'putting back' the hormones that are lost during the menopause. The body is no longer manufacturing its own supplies, but, by taking a supplement of progesterone and oestrogen – in the form of tablets, injections or even a sticky patch – you can keep your body in the standard to which it has become accustomed. The treatment is suitable for nearly all women and can be carried on as long into old age as you wish.

Where the uterus is still in place (if, for example, you have been treated with radiotherapy), the treatment consists of a balance of oestrogen and progesterone hormones, which are taken in sequence. The dose of hormone is very much smaller than that of the Pill. It is available in the form of a sticky patch, which needs changing only twice a week, and which, stuck to the thigh or buttock, allows the absorption of the hormone through the skin. But the most popular form of HRT is in Prempak-C pop-out calendar packets of pills.

If you have already passed the menopause and have had a hysterectomy, you will be prescribed oestrogen-only HRT, which has a lot of advantages for the postmenopausal woman. Oestrogen, you will recall, is the up-beat hormone and is not associated with the headaches and migraines that can become a problem for some women who are taking combined HRT. It also prevents the onset of osteoporosis, and helps to lubricate a vagina that, without HRT, may be feeling dry and sore after the menopause.

Your questions answered

Q. How can HRT prevent osteoporosis?

A. Osteoporosis is the slow process of bone thinning that makes bones brittle and susceptible to fractures. It also causes the spine to shrink, and many women lose several centimetres in height before the age of 70. Bone decay cannot be reversed, but it can be halted, and even prevented, if treatment is started early enough.

Medical research shows that a lack of the hormone oestrogen is the main cause of bone thinning. And, although calcium is also helpful, no amount of extra calcium will protect bones if the body is lacking in oestrogen. Ideally, HRT should be started as soon as possible after the onset of menopausal symptoms – irregular periods, hot flushes, sleeplessness and irritability – to prevent thinning from setting in.

Q. Will HRT make me feel as if I am pregnant?

A. In the first few months, as the body adjusts to HRT, some women experience tender breasts, nausea and leg cramps. Others report mild fluid retention and slight abdominal bloating. But these symptoms usually disappear within a matter of weeks. The average daily dose of the pregnancy hormone progesterone is only 550 units on HRT, compared to up to 5000 units received in pregnancy.

Q. I like to go swimming every day. Will I be able to use an HRT sticky patch in the pool?

A. Good for you! Swimming is excellent exercise, which, combined with HRT, will keep your body fit and prevent the onset of osteoporosis. You should have no problems with your sticky patch, as the adhesive is very strong and is the kind used on colostomy bags! Bathing and showering are also fine. But, if you are at all concerned about losing your patch in the pool, HRT tablets might be the answer for you.

Q. Will HRT improve my sex life?

A. It can do. At menopause many women lose interest in sex because the lining of the vagina dries out, and intercourse becomes painful. Replacing hormones can overcome this problem – and intercourse may even become a pleasure for the first time in many years! Especially as you won't have to worry about pregnancy.

Personal experiences of hysterectomy

DONNA'S STORY
Donna, 33, learned she had invasive cancer of the cervix at the age of 27, during her postnatal check-up after the birth of her little girl.

'Having read up a great deal about cancer, I now feel sure that I already had a tumour before becoming pregnant with Jessica, and that my pregnancy accelerated its growth. I'd had a smear in pregnancy, but the result never reached me. Somehow it got lost in the system, and, in a way, I'm pleased it did, because I would have been faced with the dilemma of whether to have treatment which could have affected Jessica.

'As it was, though, it came as a total shock to discover I had cancer when I did. I'd been bleeding a lot, but I thought it was normal post-partum bleeding that all women experience when they've had a baby.

'I was referred to St Bartholomew's Hospital, where I was told I'd need a hysterectomy. They like to keep the ovaries whenever possible, but one of mine had to be removed because the cancer had spread to the lymph on that side.

'Knowing I was in for a hysterectomy didn't bother me. All I wanted then was to get rid of the tumour. But I was totally unprepared for the terrible problems I had after the operation, trying to come to terms with losing my womb at the age of 27.

'Maybe I wouldn't have wanted another baby. But now that option had been taken away.

'Other people who didn't know what I'd been through inevitably started asking when Jessica was going to have a little brother or sister and it was difficult to explain that I couldn't have another baby because I'd had cancer and a hysterectomy.

'I also suffered a terrible blow to my self-esteem. My body image was badly affected by the operation. I had terrible scars on my stomach and felt like a freak.

'My operation had been followed with external radiotherapy. This wasn't as bad as descriptions I've heard of internal radiotherapy: my vagina hasn't been frazzled, and everything still works more or less normally. But I did experience a lot of diarrhoea during treatment, and had to time my journey back home from the hospital so I wouldn't be out of sight of a toilet at the wrong time.

'Sexually, my problems were psychological more than physical and they were exacerbated by the fact that I was a single mum and had no long-term partner to turn to for support when I was in my crisis. I thought I'd never find anyone to love me the way I was. . . . But, six years on, I have found a very loving partner who has managed to erase all those negative feelings I had about myself.

'Three years after my hysterectomy, I had to have my remaining ovary removed when it became affected with a cyst. That, I found, was far worse than the original hysterectomy. Overnight I became menopausal – going from cool, calm and collected to a raving monster. As I understand it, the surgical menopause is worse than a natural one.

'I was put on HRT, and that keeps me under control. I soon notice the change in myself if I forget to take my tablets – I immediately become irritable and unpleasant.

'Having brushed with cancer, I now look at Jessica and think how lucky I am to have her. My priorities in life have totally changed since being sick. I used to be very selfish – I'd do exactly what I wanted all the time and really did believe that cancer was something that happened to other, older women and not to someone like me. Now I have given up work to study psychology and spend more time with Jessica. We don't have all the material things I used to want, but these days I can see that there's more to life than buying things. You can't take them with you when you die. And, though I no longer see dying as an immediate possibility, I have learned about the importance of valuing my life with Jessica while I have it.'

SUE'S STORY

Sue was 25 years old and hadn't had a chance to start a family when she had a hysterectomy. Her reaction is very rare, but shows the extremes some women can experience.

'I didn't give the operation much thought at all before going into hospital. I think I actually blocked out what was happening to me.

'It was only afterwards that I reacted – in the most terrible way imaginable.

'For the first nine months, I really believed I was pregnant – because I wasn't having periods any more – and, although this sounds very silly now, I convinced myself that my husband, Charlie, had paid the doctors to impregnate me – by test tube.

'I thought that, when I eventually went into labour, Charlie would say "Surprise! We're having a baby!"

'Before losing my womb I hadn't had that sense of longing for a child. But now that the possibility of ever giving birth had been well and truly taken away from me, I yearned for motherhood.

'Ten months passed, and I realized that, no, Charlie couldn't have paid the doctors to give me a baby after all. But the grief was still there and even worse in many ways, because now I had to face up to the fact that there really was never going to be a baby.

'For a while I resorted to stuffing cushions up my dress when I went out because I wanted to look pregnant like all the other women I seemed to pass in the street.

'Everyone in the world appeared to be pregnant, and that was very painful and hard to take. The final straw came when my sister got pregnant. She wanted so desperately to share her pregnancy with me, but I wouldn't have anything to do with her. Looking back, I avoided her so successfully that I can't remember her ever having been pregnant.

'Eventually she cornered me, after the baby was born, and said, "Sue, you're killing me. You're hurting me so much." And then I had to start facing up to what I was doing and the effect my hysterectomy had had on me.

'Shortly after that, Charlie and I were listening to music together one evening and there was a couple singing to each other about their love.

'When the man sang, "Let's go and make a family together", I just felt as if I'd been punched on the nose. I totally fell apart, and was a complete wreck for weeks.

'The good thing to come out of this miserable time was that I slowed down and started grieving properly, the way I had to in order to get better.

'I began to take one day at a time and not to expect too much of myself. I went back to work – which helped, because it kept my mind occupied. But, when I felt down, I didn't try to fight it, I just went off and had a quiet cry, and came back feeling a whole lot better.

'Early on I'd always said that if I couldn't have a child of my own I didn't want one at all. But after about three years, Charlie could see that I was still very sad and unfulfilled without a baby. We'd filled the hole in our lives with exotic holidays, home improvements and lots of time together. . . . But the hole kept on getting bigger and eventually Charlie suggested adoption.

'Now we have a gorgeous little boy called Stephen. I feel as if he's my very own, and I'm so happy that I can't even remember what life was like without him.'

ROZ'S STORY
Roz, 41, was 34 when she had a total hysterectomy.

'I'd been referred for a cone biopsy after the discovery of CIN 3 cells on my smear test. But the cells were so deep that the surgeon couldn't get a clear margin around the section he'd removed, so the next step was a hysterectomy.

'I didn't have any children and, at that point, hadn't ever planned to have them, but it did occur to me that this might be a problem for me after the operation. I wondered whether, once I'd lost my womb, I'd regret the fact that having a family was no longer an option.

'In fact, I had none of these normal psychological problems and my physical recovery was brilliant, too. The doctors said I broke all records for speed of recovery after the operation – and they said that was because I'd prepared myself so well prior to surgery.

'I had seven weeks' notice that I was going into hospital, and I deliberately set out to get as fit as I possibly could. I swam regularly, took a lot of fitness classes, and made sure my diet was really healthy. I'd also read, stitch for stitch, what was involved in the operation, so when I woke up with various tubes attached to me I knew exactly what each one was for.

'I'd read that wind is a major problem after hysterectomy and, for that reason, I ate hardly anything for two days before surgery – and this helped a great deal.

'I didn't have any pain after the operation, just a dragging feeling if I stood still – say peeling potatoes or doing the washing-up – for any length of time. Walking around was fine though.

'The biggest problem with me was that I couldn't believe I'd really had those CIN 3 cells. I felt as fit as a fiddle and kept expecting someone to come and say, "Sorry love, we got it wrong. You weren't the one with the abnormal smear." But of course, nobody ever did say that, and, since having the hysterectomy, I have become quite paranoid about my health – imagining every lump and bump to be cancer.

'The good thing about this, though, is that it means I take enormous care of myself now. I eat loads of fresh fruit and vegetables, and keep up with my fitness regime. I've learned that you can't take your good health for granted.'

LOUISE'S STORY

Louise was 31 and expecting her third baby when she had a positive smear, 12 years ago.

'Like many women getting that news, I was really scared I would die and wouldn't be around for the children. And that fear increased when my doctor discovered that the cone biopsy I'd had to treat my CIN 3 hadn't worked. I was told I'd need a hysterectomy, but I was beginning to lose faith in medicine and wondered whether this would work since the cone biopsy hadn't.

'But that fear focused my mind and made me really take good care to look after myself. The thing that upset me most about the hysterectomy was the loss of femininity that went with it. Having just had three children, I was at that stage we all go through when I wasn't bothering so much with make-up and I'd happily slop around in a pair of jeans and a sweatshirt. But, suddenly, I was horrified by the prospect of (I imagined) becoming fat, hairy and unattractive with the loss of my womb.

'So, as soon as I was up to it, I booked some keep-fit classes, had my hair cut and invested in some new clothes and make-up.

'I'm a very positive person – always looking on the bright side of any situation – and having had that brush with cancer, which reminds you that nothing is certain in life, I started taking every opportunity that came along. Instead of sitting at home feeling sorry for myself, I was out and about, doing things with the kids, but also getting on with my own career and interests. I didn't put things off any more. It's no good thinking I'll do that when I'm older – none of us knows whether we will be there when that "older" time comes!

'I also made sure I wasn't horrible to people – my experience taught me to value friends and family too, and not to take them for granted.

'I'd kept my ovaries so I didn't have to contend with the hormonal changes some women undergo after hysterectomy. I've been told there's more possibility menopause will strike early after what I've been through, but it doesn't worry me, because I know that HRT is there to cushion the fall.'

Your sexuality after hysterectomy

The ways in which hysterectomy affects a woman's sexuality and her enjoyment of sex vary enormously. Some women report that their G spot appears to have been removed along with everything else. While it is unlikely this has happened, it is possible that the G spot has moved – and has not yet been relocated! – or that reduced sensation elsewhere in the vagina seems to have impaired the feelings around the G spot.

There is also the problem, for a lot of women who enjoy uterine and cervical contractions as part of their orgasm, that orgasms are now not possible in the way they used to be. But, even if this is the case, all is not lost. It is possible, with the help of a supportive partner and a sympathetic sexual therapist, to 'restructure' lovemaking so that you gain more pleasure from areas you had not previously explored. For women whose orgasms are mainly clitoral, losing the uterus is less of a problem. And for those who have been used to widespreading reverberations, concentrating more on clitoral pleasure – along with other erogenous zones – can prove very fulfilling.

So, for some women a hysterectomy provides new pleasures in their sex life. While for others, sex after a hysterectomy actually becomes more enjoyable than ever before. Sue says:

> Sex has been a very fulfilling part of my life since having my hysterectomy. I'd suffered endometriosis for years before the operation, and it had made intercourse extremely painful. Now I feel totally liberated. I orgasm easily, something which I never managed before, and my orgasms are very intense and satisfying.

Angela adds:

> After 20 years of pain during intercourse, I was eager to discover whether there had been any improvement after my hysterectomy. The surgeon warned me not to attempt intercourse until I'd seen him for my post-op check-up. But when the day eventually came, I saw him at the clinic in the afternoon, and, that evening, my husband and I made love – albeit in a rush. After the initial panic, we slowed down and found to our delight that I had no pain in any

position. Just sheer joy and multiple orgasms on almost every occasion. Things are still going well and we are both extremely happy with our love life.

If you experience sexual problems after hysterectomy, do not assume that this is the way things are going to be from now on – it is not your lot to have to put up with a diminished sex life and, in fact, the more you have sex, the more good you will be doing yourself because regular sexual activity encourages the vagina to stay elastic and comfortable.

That said, painful sex – for reasons that may be physical or psychological – is not going to whet the appetite for more of the same. And the more you avoid sex, the more your vagina will atrophy (as these changes are called). So sex becomes more painful the less you try.

If you have the kind of doctor who is dismissive of these kinds of worries, try to find someone else you can talk to who may be better placed to help. If there is a MacMillan nurse attached to your ward at the hospital, she will be able to help you discuss your problems. So, too, will a sexual therapist at a couples' counselling centre like Relate. Hysterectomy is unlikely to leave you feeling like the person you were before the operation, but do not assume that just because you are now different, you are worse off than before. Suzie Hayman points out that orgasms after hysterectomy are often found to be sharper and more intense in sensation. Your feelings can be localized on your clitoris, rather than diffused and spread out. For this reason some women say the experience is even more gratifying.

7

Why me? What causes cervical cancer?

LIZ'S STORY

Liz has never received any treatment for pre-cancer or cancer of the cervix. But, at the age of 31, she has been warned that her smear has shown up borderline changes, which are now being regularly checked in case of any deterioration.

'When I asked the doctor what could have caused these changes, she said it was possibly the human papilloma (wart) virus, and that I may have caught it from my husband.

'That knowledge has badly affected our sex life. He's the only partner I have ever had. But I know he'd had partners before me and I worry that, if he has the virus, I might be putting myself in greater risk by continuing to sleep with him.

'I've lost all interest in him now, because I just see him as a risk, a threat to my life. Things are so bad that we have made an appointment to see a sex therapist, because, somehow, I've got to get rid of this terrible image of him that I've built up.

REBECCA'S STORY CONTINUED

After having treatment for cancer of the cervix, Rebecca is finding sexual intercourse physically impossible. But there is also a psychological problem.

'Although I've only ever had one partner, I know my husband slept with other women before meeting me.

'Now I worry that, if I developed cancer once and sex is one of the causes, then, by having sex, I am putting myself in the same danger again.

'My husband and I talk about the physical aspects, and he promises me he understands how I feel. But then he asks why I don't use my dilators, and that shows he doesn't really understand at all.

'I asked my radiotherapist why nobody thought of testing husbands to see if they had HPV, but he said that would open too many cans of worms.'

And, besides, testing husbands does not solve the wife's cancer. It is true that cervical cancer has the potential to open up a can of worms. Once a sexual link has been identified, some women blame their partners, others blame themselves. They suffer guilt, anxiety and feelings that they are being punished. They may feel dirty and contaminated.

But how realistic are these feelings, and how rational is it to assume that a sexual trigger led to the disease in the first place, so it might do the same again?

There are two types of cervical cancer.

Squamous – which is by far the most common type of cervical cancer, and almost certainly the result of some process that occurs during sexual intercourse. A link with HPV is strongly indicated, and a woman having a sexual relationship with a man who has genital warts has about a one in three risk of developing a pre-cancerous condition of the cervix.

Adenocarcinoma – which is the much rarer form of cervical cancer, can affect women who have never had sexual intercourse.

Therefore, not all cervical cancer is caused by sexual intercourse.

The sexual link

There is a lot of evidence pointing to the fact that some men are carriers of agents that trigger cervical cancer in their partners.

- A high protein content in semen may cause changes in the cervical skin that can progress to pre-cancer. One theory is that a substance in the protein of certain high-risk men's semen can be harmful when it comes into contact with an unformed, maturing cervix.

Another theory is that substances in the seminal fluid, which carries the sperm and which is necessary to allow fertilization of a woman's egg, may reduce her ability to overcome the disease. If this is the case, a woman's chances of developing cervical cancer are increased by having unprotected sexual intercourse.

- The human papilloma virus (HPV) was first identified as a cause in the late 1970s. Some men will know that they have HPV because the warts on their penis are obvious. Where they are so evident, they can be easily treated with laser treatment or a paint-on ointment, like podophyllin, which burns the wart off.

However, many men may be unaware that they have the wart virus, because the warts are too small to be seen with the naked eye. Also, warts are not something they can easily control. Certainly a man wouldn't set out to have warts and infect his partner with the virus that caused them, so, although we may be tempted to blame men for the part they play here, it is neither logical nor reasonable to do so (See Your questions answered, page 72). As the wart virus can be transferred from women to uninfected men, the more partners a man has, the more likely he is to become infected with the virus.

- Exposure to certain chemicals at work can also increase a man's likelihood of introducing pre-cancerous changes to his partner. Studies have shown a link between so-called dirty jobs and a higher incidence of positive smears in women workers or the female partners of male workers. Chemicals once absorbed into the body can appear in traces in the semen, or on the genitals.

- The partners of men who smoke have also been shown to be at increased risk of cervical cancer. But a woman who smokes is at even greater risk.

There have been a number of cases reported where, with a little bit of detective work, the sexual link has been identified and traced back to a sexual partner and his past girlfriends. One example is a woman who had her first positive smear just after embarking on her second ever sexual relationship. Her doctor discovered that the woman's new partner's first wife had also been treated for the disease. So, it seems, men can definitely play a part in introducing pre-cancer or CIN.

What other sexual causes, or promoters, have been suggested?

- The younger a woman is when she becomes sexually active, the greater the risk of developing cervical cancer. This is because, when we are young, the cells of our cervix are immature. They mature as we grow older, and become more capable of withstanding the processes resulting from the effects of sexual penetration. Exposure to these processes before maturation has taken place can damage these delicate cells. Some studies suggest that having intercourse under the age of 21 poses the greatest risk.

- The more male partners a woman has, the more chance she has of developing cancer, because there is a greater risk of her coming into contact with the trigger agent contained in the wart which causes cancer.

- The earlier a woman has her first child, the more vulnerable she is because, again, the cervix is not fully mature and may suffer cell damage in the process of childbirth.

- The Pill is the most reliable form of contraception available for most of us. However, it can reduce our natural immunity to infection and can also affect the way we use folic acid (and there is some evidence to suggest that women with positive smears often have a folic acid deficiency). By using the Pill, we are also less likely to use a barrier method, which, as well as protecting against pregnancy, protects us from infection and disease. However, the Pill significantly reduces ovarian cancer, which is a much bigger killer.

Non-sexual factors

Diet

A poor diet – one that is lacking in fresh fruit and vegetables, fish and energy rich pastas and pulses, but high in fat, caffeine and alcohol – increases your vulnerability to disease of any kind. Deficiencies in vitamin C, beta carotene and folic acid also put us at risk of becoming ill.

Smoking

Carcinogens show up in your cervical secretions in ten times the quantity they do in your blood, so smoking 20 cigarettes a day makes you 7 times more vulnerable to cancer, and 40 a day increases your vulnerability to 14 times that of a non-smoker. The nicotine in cigarettes gets into your mucus covering the cervix, lowering your cervical cells' natural resistance to abnormal changes and, because smoking generally lowers your immune system, you are really attacking yourself from all sides.

If you have had a positive smear, you should stop smoking.

Stress

Stress inhibits our ability to throw off ill-health, and is always mentioned in connection with cancer. This is because when we are under stress, our normal healthy resistance is lowered and our cells are more vulnerable to disease. Jane Metcalfe, co-author of *The Bristol Experience*, was diagnosed as having cervical cancer six years ago. She says:

> I wasn't really surprised. I had experienced a great deal of stress in my life over the three years leading up to my diagnosis.
>
> I was an opera singer – a job which sounds wonderful to outsiders but is, in fact, very competitive and high-pressured. I used to swing between depression when things weren't going well, and elation when they were. Those extreme highs and lows can be very hard to handle.
>
> On top of this I was in a marriage which was crumbling because of financial difficulties. We had a baby boy who never slept, so I spent the first three years of his life in a constant state of exhaustion.
>
> My marriage finally broke up – and then started a custody battle over our son, resulting in even more stress, and, on top of all this, I was still struggling to keep my career afloat.
>
> It's not surprising my health broke down, but when the cancer was finally diagnosed (see Jane's story in Chapter 1), in some ways it was almost a relief because it gave me the opportunity to take stock of my life and make a new start.

Making sure the same thing doesn't happen again

If you have had a positive smear and received treatment, there is no reason to believe you will become infected with whatever trigger caused your cell changes the first time round because you are now in a better position than before to understand the causes and to avoid them.

That does not mean avoiding sex like Liz and Rebecca. Instead, think about protected sex, and, if there's a physical problem as well, consider talking to a psycho-sexual therapist about ways in which you can enjoy non-penetrative sex.

If you live in a polluted environment, smoke or follow a bad diet, look at ways in which you can improve your quality of life.

In the next chapter we will be looking at self-help in treating cancer, and also preventative tactics to employ against the disease.

Your questions answered

Q. I have just discovered that my present partner's last girlfriend had cervical cancer. Does that mean I am at risk too?

A. There is evidence which shows that if a man has sexual intercourse with a woman who has cervical cancer or pre-cancer, his subsequent sexual partners may also develop the disease. If your partner's last girlfriend has had cervical cancer, there is a strong possibility that she developed this as a result of having the human papilloma (wart) virus. Even if she did not catch the warts from your partner, during the course of their relationship, he may have caught them from her. This is something you should discuss with your doctor, who may recommend that you have smears more regularly than once every three or five years. Regular smears will show not only whether you have pre-cancer, but whether you have warts. But you should also use a condom for added protection during intercourse.

Q. How can I find out if my new partner has HPV?

A. Warts on the penis are not necessarily cancer-causing, but because tests to identify the types of virus they contain are complicated and expensive, it is safer to assume that anyone with visible warts is a high-risk partner. Not all warts are obvious to the human eye, however, and those that aren't can only be detected under colposcopic examination, but this screening is rarely performed.

Q. If all strains of HPV are not cancer-causing, what is the probability of coming into contact with one that is?

A. There are currently over 72 different types of wart virus, but the number is constantly growing as more are identified. Not all of them cause cancer, but high-risk and low-risk warts are capable of living side by side. Studies suggest that half of the female population have come into contact with harmful (cancer-causing) wart viruses at some time in their life. But not everyone holds on to the virus – you can shake it off the way you shake off any other germs. Only those who do keep the virus (and you are more at risk if you smoke and have a poor diet) are at risk of developing this form of cancer, and, even then, not every woman with the wart virus will necessarily contract cancer.

Q. My husband has a wart on his finger – could that cause cervical cancer?

A. No – this isn't possible. Although the kinds of warts that appear on fingers are caused by HPV, this is not the same strain as the HPV that causes genital warts and cancer. There is absolutely no risk of a finger wart harming your cervix.

Q. My husband claims he has only ever slept with me. Now I have a positive smear, does it mean he has been lying to me? Could he have got HPV without having another sexual partner?

A. Don't judge your husband too harshly – it's just possible he's telling the truth! First, although scientists expect genital warts to be transmitted sexually, they are still looking into the possibility that some men have developed them without sexual transmission.

Second, remember that there are two types of cervical cancer. The rarer type, adenocarcinoma, is *not* sexually transmitted and has been found in virgins – and it's possible your CIN changes are linked to this type of cancer.

8

Self-help – a positive approach

Most of us, however open we are to the idea of treating ourselves with home remedies for coughs, colds or flu, would shudder at the prospect of single-handedly taking on an illness as serious as cancer.

However, without exception, the women who have told their stories in this book have had the fighting spirit to read up about their CIN or cancer, to try to understand what is happening to their body, and to ask, 'Is this the right treatment for me?', and, 'What are the alternatives?'

For some, the questions come too late. It is only in retrospect that you wish you'd had the guts to ask questions about your illness and its treatment. For others, it was their positive attitude that secured them the treatment of their choice.

Winifred explained (on page 32) how she read up and researched all she could about her CIN changes before choosing to pay a private doctor for loop diathermy treatment. In the course of her research, she also looked into ways of preventing the abnormal cells from recurring.

I'd been on the Pill since my early twenties and was interested to read that the Pill can deplete our natural stores of folic acid. A folic acid deficiency, in turn, can encourage the development of pre-cancerous cells.

I also read that vitamin C and E deficiency can make a person more vulnerable to cancer.

Since being treated for CIN, I have changed the whole family's diet so we now eat more fresh fruit and vegetables – at least five portions each per day. And I also use vitamin C and E and folic acid supplements.

Apart from knowing that I'm actively helping my body fight any new cancer cells which may try to develop in the future, I've never felt better in my life!

The self-help I am recommending in this chapter is *complementary* rather than *alternative*. It is advice on lifestyle changes you can make alongside conventional treatment, which will help you understand and put your cancer in perspective, and, hopefully, alleviate some of the symptoms. In many cases it can also help to speed up your cure.

The main changes you should aim to make are:

- to learn to relax
- to improve your diet.

Stress lowers the body's resistance and encourages the growth of cancer. Learning to relax and switch off from stress will slow down, or stem, the process. Diet is important, too, because poor nutrition is reported to be at the core of at least a third of all cancers, and, in studies, women with positive smears have been discovered to have diets containing less than 30 mg of vitamin C a day.

You should also learn to talk about your pre-cancer and your fears concerning it.

Several studies have shown a link between cancer and personality, though this idea is poo-pooed by a lot of people who have cancer as well as those who treat it. The holistic practitioner Laurence LeShan lists the following as being characteristics of a typical 'cancer personality':

- unsettled childhood
- low opinion of yourself
- unsatisfactory relationship with your parents
- no creative outlets
- keeping a tight lid on your emotions
- a defeatist attitude
- loss of an important relationship.

What may be true, however, of almost anyone who has cancer, is that talking about it does not come easily. Certainly many of the women I spoke to about cervical cancer, or even straightforward abnormal smears, found this an embarrassing subject to raise in conversation.

And, as Liz Hodgkinson, co-author with Jane Metcalfe of *The Bristol Experience*, points out, although statistics tell us that one in three people get cancer, most new patients realize that they don't know anyone else in the world who has the illness. And they don't know where to turn to.

Talking your own problems through

Cancer self-help and support groups, such as those run by the charity CancerLink (for their address, see the Useful addresses section at the back of the book), can be a great starting point for opening up and talking about the complex of emotions you are having to contend with alongside your illness. A counsellor can also be a tremendous help.

Groups work on the principle that a problem shared is a problem halved, and that does seem to help many people to cope with the isolation and depression that accompany cancer. Counselling helps further by allowing you as an individual to open up and explore every emotion with the help of a skilled therapist who, unlike friends and family members, will not take exception to, or become upset by, any of the feelings you reveal.

Both group therapy and counselling can help your partner and family to cope with the difficult emotions they are also having to deal with.

For all of you, though, there will be the problem of what to tell your children. And I'd like to offer some advice here, based on information issued by the American Cancer Society for helping children cope when a parent has cancer.

Talking with your children

A good friend of mine lost her mother to cancer when she was just eight years old. She knew her mother was ill – but did not know exactly what was wrong with her – and she says she had no idea that her mother was dying:

> She was there, ill in her bed on the Friday when I was packed off to stay with my grandparents. But, when I was brought back, on the Monday, she was gone.

This memory still torments Angela in adulthood. And while most of us now know that it is wrong to ignore a child's feelings at a traumatic time like this, it can still be difficult to know exactly how to tell them what is going on.

Children have five basic needs.

- Information – let your children say what's on their minds, and be receptive to any questions they have about your illness and treatment. Children need to know that parents and other adults are there to think things through with them.
- Emotional support – above all else, children need to feel loved and cared for. Keeping up with their usual routines as much as possible will show them that they still matter very much to you. They may also need encouragement in expressing feelings of fear, anger, guilt and sadness. Just like adults, children find ways of protecting themselves from these feelings. Help them understand that their emotions are normal and show them it's important to let their feelings out.
- Responsibilities and choices – give your children opportunities to do things that make them feel they are helping you – fetching you a glass of water or reading to you, for example. And let them know they have a choice in what they do. Don't make decisions for them. Instead, ask, 'Do you want to visit at hospital, or stay at home with Grandma?' Choices and responsibilities give children the feeling we all benefit from, of being in control.
- Breathing space – especially if your child is becoming too adult-like, doing the housework, etc., to compensate for your own withdrawal from certain domestic activities, make sure they have time off for fun – with their friends and also with the whole family.
- Hope – every member of a family experiencing cancer lives with uncertainty and many children worry about what the future holds. A clear understanding of what is happening, and the reassurance that they will be loved and cared for *regardless* of what happens, is vital at this difficult time. Make sure they know, too, that a lot of the side-effects of your treatment or stay in hospital are temporary.

Is there a natural treatment for CIN?

If you are really set against conventional medical treatment, alternatives such as herbalism are also available.

DENISE'S STORY

Denise was 25 and her baby daughter was 3 months old when she had her first ever positive smear a year ago. The doctor told her she had CIN 2 cells, and urged her to go to hospital for a further investigation.

'I wasn't at all keen on this idea. I'd just had a traumatic time giving birth in the same hospital – I'd been whipped in for a Caesarean after months of carefully planning a home birth. I'd also read that hormonal changes after the birth of a baby can cause cell changes in the cervix, so I wasn't convinced the condition was pre-cancerous, and asked the doctor to repeat the test.

'When she refused, I went to a private clinic for a smear. In fact, this result told me the cells were CIN 3. But, still convinced that the changes were something to do with the birth of my baby, and because I fitted into none of the risk factors – neither my husband nor I have ever been promiscuous, we don't smoke, we eat a healthy vegan diet, and we live in the countryside so we're not affected by pollution – I decided to find an alternative to conventional treatment.

'I found a herbalist who had treated CIN 1 and 2 with success, but I was her first CIN 3, so I was something of a test case.

'The treatment was very involved: I had to travel for six hours on my return journeys to see her, and I had to do this twice a week for nine weeks. She talked to me and treated me as a whole person, not just a cervix, and gave me herbal douches and pessaries, which I used every day. I also took vitamin supplements and followed a vegan diet.

'We got around to talking about the belief which many alternative practitioners hold that a trauma to a certain part of the body can produce a block of the body's Ch'i energy in this place.

'It occurred to us both, knowing my history, that my cervix could have responded to the shock of a Caesarean section when it had been preparing for birth. And even if this was not the case, there was still the possibility that breastfeeding had brought about a hormonal change.

'I had millions of cards sent to me urging me to attend the colposcopy clinic for treatment. I refused to do this, but did agree to a biopsy so I could monitor the advance of the rogue cells.

The first biopsy came back with a CIN 3 result. But I was still only halfway through my herbal cure, so I decided to give it a few more weeks.

'Eight weeks later I had another biopsy and by this time had decided that, if CIN 3 was still present, I would have the cells removed with loop diathermy.

'The colposcopist was convinced I was wasting my time even thinking that this wouldn't be the outcome. But her face brightened amazingly when she looked at my cervix, and she said, "Oh, that's looking much better!" She sent me away to see if the cells cleared up any further, and, when I went back for a follow-up biopsy two months' later, the results showed I was completely clear . . . !'

In America, naturopathic cervical escarotic treatment – a form of herbalism – is quite widely used by naturopathic doctors for the treatment of CIN 1 and CIN 2 – and it has good success rates. As doctors in the United States work closely with gynaecologists it is easy to get the treatment you want. In the UK it is not so easy to find a herbalist who has experience of treating pre-cancerous conditions, and, when you do, you may have some difficulty persuading your gynaecologist to work alongside the herbal practitioner. However, the National Institute of Medical Herbalists (see Useful addresses) should be able to put you in touch with herbalists in your area, and, by a process of elimination, you should, with luck, find someone able to help you.

Your herbalist will recommend that you continue to keep up all your investigative appointments with the gynaecology department, and it is important that you do this in order to monitor the progress of your abnormal cells and to be certain that the condition is not becoming more severe.

Naturopathic cervical escarotic treatment uses local treatments on the abnormal cells, usually in the form of douches or pessaries. Your practitioner will also give you treatments to boost your immune system and help you fight the possible onset of cancer.

For inflammatory pre-CIN changes, a herbalist may suggest you use diluted calendula (marigold, which is a classic anti-inflammatory preparation) in water as a douche. For CIN 1 and 2, the calendula might be mixed with tinctures of thuja (tree of life). Do seek professional advice from a herbalist and *never attempt to make your own treatments*.

DENISE'S STORY CONTINUED

'There were times when I felt everyone was against me. Locally, people thought I was mad not to go along with conventional medicine. They were all convinced I was laying myself open to get full-blown cancer. The doctors were appalled too by what they saw as my cavalier attitude to the disease. They didn't understand that, for me, conventional medicine seems invasive and harmful, and I was therefore doing my very best for my health by working closely with a herbalist to treat my CIN 3.

'I'd said all along that if, after the herbal treatment had finished, there was no improvement, I would do what the gynaecologist recommended. But I wanted to give myself a chance, first, of what I saw as a healthy cure.

'When the biopsy results finally came through showing no trace of abnormal cells, the doctor refused to believe it was true. "This kind of thing just doesn't happen," he said. "You've gone untreated – the cells must still be dyskaryotic."

' "But I have been treated," I insisted. "I've been using herbal treatments."

' "Oh, yes," he grunted. "I've heard all about that!" '

Complementary approaches to cancer

There are over 200 complementary therapies, ranging from aroma-therapy to meditation. And what all of them aim to do is to look not just at your cervix and why it has CIN or cancer, but at you as a whole person, and to ask, 'Why has this person got cancer?'

Colin Ryder Richardson, Director of the charity New Approaches to Cancer, believes the answer to this question nearly always has to do with the kind of person that you are. He believes there is definitely a 'cancer personality' and it is generally the kind of person who puts other people before herself.

While doctors do not agree with many of Colin's views, he

believes that:

> Ninety per cent of cancer is stress. You only have to look at today's society to see why that is. Marriage, trust, etc. are all going out of the window – and stress is rising. People who develop cancer have often suffered a lot of guilt, self-blame and general fretting, and all this negativity eventually implodes on themselves, making them very sick. They have to learn to look after number one before they can treat their cancer – and the way to do this is through complementary approaches which nurture them and make them feel more secure, lovable and at ease with themselves.

There isn't room here to go into all 200 therapies, but let's look at some of the most important ones being used by the Bristol Cancer Help Centre.

Circle dancing

This may sound like an odd form of therapy, but, for Jane Metcalfe, it became a favourite when she was at the Bristol Centre. It involves very simple steps, done while standing as part of a group in a circle, and Jane says, 'it brings profound emotions to the surface and allows them to be harmlessly dispelled. You can't help but smile, and the activity enables sadness to be danced away.'

Diet

There is, as I've already outlined, a definite link between diet and cancer. But recommendations for the kind of diet we should follow to combat the disease vary enormously.

In general though, the guidelines for a healthy anti-cancer diet are these – eat:

- plenty of fresh fruit and vegetables, preferably organic and raw, but, if necessary, very lightly steamed (as soon as the cooking starts, the vitamins are lost)
- little or no animal products
- plenty of vitamins C and E, beta carotene and folic acid
- no sugar, fat, salt, spices or caffeine.

Why? Because salt contains a lot of sodium chloride, which tends to deplete levels of potassium, which healthy cells need to function at full capacity. Sugar is generally bad for you – as you have been told from childhood – very addictive and contains empty calories. And caffeine stimulates adrenalin production and gives you a hyped-up feeling. It also dilates blood vessels and encourages carcinogenic substances, known as nitrosamines, to form in the stomach.

How easy is it to have a balanced meal without meat, cheese, fish, salt, spices or sugar? Very easy!

Even a baked potato served with humus and a salad makes a nutritionally well-balanced and Bristol-approved meal that the whole family can enjoy.

Colin Ryder Richardson says:

You can also tell how healthy your diet is by examining what comes out when you go to the loo. If your elimination is good, your diet is healthy. If it is bad, and you are constipated, there are all sorts of horrid toxins sitting in your bowel which isn't at all healthy.

(Following treatment for cancer, it is usual to have bowel changes such as constipation, regardless of your diet, so don't worry unnecessarily!)

Massage and shiatsu

Especially if you have had radiotherapy treatment or hysterectomy that has knocked your self-esteem and left you with a poor body image, you may be tempted to run at the prospect of lying naked while someone touches you. But masseurs are used to working with all types of bodies, and, after a few treatments, you will start to enjoy the 'hands on' contact and start loving your body again – so massage is very valuable to anyone who feels sad, unattractive and unlovable during or after their illness.

Shiatsu is particularly good for cancer patients because it focuses on areas of the skin known as pressure points, where the body's vital Ch'i energy is strongest. The idea is that, as these points are touched, energy that has previously been blocked starts to flow again.

Unlike massage, which tends to be done when the patient is naked or in her underwear, shiatsu is done through clothes and it is not just surface treatment – its aim is to release stress and pent-up anxiety and to balance the body.

Meditation

Meditation is, Colin Ryder Richardson explains, the ability to enter an altered state of mind. At its best, it can enable you to travel in your mind so that you are sitting in the Himalayas or on a beach in the South of France – 'Who needs holidays when you can go where you like, when you like, in your mind?', he says.

In practice, though, many people find meditation extremely difficult. Especially when you are wound up and tense, it can be impossible to concentrate on one thought to the exclusion of all others and boring to focus on a candle flame (a popular image) for five minutes. But meditation has always been considered important at the Bristol Cancer Help Centre, and, with practice, patients can learn to use it to escape, like escaping into an oasis, at different times of the day when life is stressful and everything seems to be getting on top of you.

Transcendental meditation can be taught on a one-to-one basis or in a group, and, in the Useful addresses section at the end of this book is an address to find out more about what is available in your area.

Music and art therapy

These are based on the belief that many of our deepest feelings are impossible to express in words, but come out quite easily through art or music. Jane Metcalfe describes the experience of one woman who went to Bristol, dreading art therapy:

> She was sure that everyone else would be an artist, and that she would be the laughing stock of the class. But nobody laughed and she soon found she could see the way she was healing through the things she painted and her efforts to perfect them.

Relaxation

Relaxation – true relaxation – is not as straightforward as many of us may think. It is not simply a matter of flopping in front of the television (which can actually accentuate our stress and play on our emotions with all the thoughts and reactions it provokes).

True relaxation comes from learning to breathe slowly and deeply, a process which enables our body and mind to wind down and become calm. Breathing and relaxation go together because you cannot breathe properly without first being relaxed. And you can't relax unless you learn to breathe deeply!

As babies, we breathe correctly – from the abdomen, the ribcage, the back and upper chest. It is only as we get older that we lose this natural knack and start, through fear and anxiety, to breathe shallowly. As we do so, we store up tension and become constantly hyped up.

Re-educating ourselves to breathe deeply in adulthood helps to alleviate the stress we feel (constantly if we are trying to cope with cancer). This, in turn, boosts the immune system (which suffers from stress). There is also a theory (although not altogether popular) that cancer cells thrive when starved of oxygen, so deep breathing has a special significance for cancer patients.

It is easier to practise deep breathing and relaxation in a group than alone, and, for many people, a yoga class is the perfect place to do this.

Spiritual healing

This is given different names by different people – if you are a Christian, you may believe in the power of prayer, otherwise you may believe in positive thinking. They amount to more or less the same thing, which is the belief that some people are able to tap into a healing force that can be chanelled from the healer to the sick person. Sometimes it involves the 'laying on of hands', but it can also be done from a distance.

Very often, it takes a crisis such as cancer to make people willing to accept spiritual healing, but it has been found to be of tremendous benefit to cancer patients. You do not have to follow any particular religious faith in order to take part in it, though those with faith may be happier seeing a practitioner who has the same beliefs.

Visualization

Most people have now heard of visualization techniques used to fight cancer. These were developed by the American cancer specialists

Carl and Stephanie Simonton, and the most famous image they have suggested is the one where the healthy white cells of the body are sharks that attack and eat all the cancerous cells, which are seen as cauliflowers.

Visualization hasn't turned out to be the star therapy it was once hailed to be, but it can be a very useful tool in all aspects of your cancer care.

In Chapter 5, Fiona told us how she used visualization to 'make friends' with her radiotherapy. Other cancer patients have used the technique to befriend their chemotherapy medicines, and even to visualize all the doctors and nurses attending them as their own close family members who only want the best for them.

At Bristol, the visualization sessions focus on the patients seeing themselves as perfect human beings – spiritually, mentally and physically. This is an idea that has a lot in common with another complementary philosophy – that of Louise Hay, author of *You Can Heal Your Life*.

Louise Hay claims she cured her cancer by changing her thoughts about herself and learning to love herself. The core of her philosophy is that our thoughts create our reality. However negative or stressful our thoughts are, they are generated from within ourselves. We choose what we think about, and by choosing to think that we are a lovely, perfect, lovable person – all over and inside, warts, hysterectomy scars and all – we gain the ability to heal ourselves and (preferably alongside conventional medicine) overcome something that is as frightening and menacing as cancer.

In conclusion

When Jane Metcalfe arrived at the Bristol Cancer Help Centre, she was asked, 'Why have you come here?'

'To cure my cancer,' she replied.

'In that case, you are setting yourself up for failure,' she was told.

Complementary therapies can help, but they are not a guaranteed cure and to think of them as such is to misunderstand what they are about.

Don't start a holistic approach to cancer *expecting* it to cure you, but, rather, use it to improve your general health, to help prevent the cancer from returning once you are in remission. Studies have shown that women who are treated for cervical cancer and then get back on with their old lives, not changing a thing, are less likely to survive than those who see their cancer as a turning point, a time to take stock of their lives and make all-round improvements.

9

All clear?

You've had the bad news that your smear was 'positive'. You've received the treatment, if necessary, recommended by your gynaecologist. You've possibly even had to cope with the 'death sentence' of cancer. Now you've come out the other side – your body is clear of malignant cells, you are free to get on with your life. But, for many women, there is an insecurity now that will never go away. Like them, you may feel you will never be the same again.

It is important to remember that even if left untreated, many cases of CIN 1 and 2 can go back to normal. Of CIN 1 cases, estimates suggest that 60 per cent will regress, 26 per cent remain exactly the same, and only 14 per cent get worse. Of this 14 per cent, only half will progress to become invasive cancer. And, although the death rates from invasive cervical cancer are a frightening 50 per cent, don't forget that 85 per cent of women who have invasive cancer have never had a smear, and most of the remaining 15 per cent have only ever attended for a single smear.

Dr Anne Szarewski, Senior Clinical Medical Officer at the Margaret Pyke Centre, says:

> Many of the women who die from cervical cancer will not have noticed anything wrong until it was too late. We must never forget the importance of regular cervical screening.

Cervical cancer is a distressing and potentially fatal disease, but, if you have been attending for regular smears and receive treatment for pre-cancerous changes, or if your cancer is found and treated at an early stage, you have a very good chance of a complete recovery.

Even so, lingering doubts are inevitable.

Roz, who told her story in Chapter 6, describes the typical emotions that rumble on for years after a brief encounter with cancer.

- Guilt

  It is impossible not to ask yourself, 'Why me? What did I do to deserve this?' However many people tell you these thoughts are irrational, it is hard not to feel guilty.

- Anger

  I'd wanted a smear test sooner than the standard five-year recall date. But my GP told me this wasn't possible. Like it or not, I had to wait my turn like every other woman. Then, when my turn came, I found I had CIN 3 changes. I was 'too advanced' for loop diathermy treatment, which would have been my treatment of choice, and had to have a cone biopsy. This didn't work, and I ended up having a hysterectomy. The lasting effect of this was sheer anger on my part that the Government is not willing to fund more regular smears and that I and many other women are put through unnecessary surgery.

  I wrote to my local MP, but never even got a reply. And, even now, I feel cross that women's health is treated so lightly.

- Denial

  At every stage up to and after my hysterectomy, I expected someone to come along and say, 'Sorry, love! We got it wrong – you didn't have an abnormal smear at all, we were looking at someone else's results'. I felt so fit and healthy that I couldn't believe I had pre-cancerous cells. And, six years on, I still have days when I think it didn't really happen.

- Fear

  You get on with your life and keep yourself as healthy as possible. But, at the back of your mind, there's always that nagging fear that something will make the cancer come back. My mother died of cancer of the bowel, which later spread to the spine, and although I am in very good health, part of me is waiting for another tumour to pop up somewhere in my body. I am sure that whatever age I am when I eventually die – be it 50 or 80 – I will die of cancer.

All these feelings are entirely normal, and there can be very few people in the world who, having brushed with cancer once, don't experience some emotional fall-out. But, when, as a result of having an abnormal smear or a diagnosis of cancer, we are forced to take a fresh look at our lives, to make more time for ourselves and to make the most of everything we have, we must surely see the cancer as having been a positive turning point. Cancer changes your life, but it doesn't have to be a change for the worse. And, as Sheena's triumph over tragedy story tells us, it can have the most amazing outcome.

SHEENA'S STORY

'I was 32 and my husband Brian and I were planning to start a family. Brian had been offered a year's teaching exchange in Canada, and we assumed that by the time we returned to England I'd be pregnant.

'But conceiving our first child was not as easy as we'd imagined. And, when we came back home, in the autumn of 1987, I asked my GP if he could help. I was referred to a consultant, who put me through a range of fertility tests and, then, early in the New Year of 1988, suggested I go in for a laparoscopy so he could see what was going on inside me.

'The next thing I knew I was being asked to go back – this time for a colposcopy. I knew this was a test used to look at the cervix and couldn't quite imagine why I was being brought in for it when I'd had no unusual symptoms – no bleeding, pain or discharge which would have suggested there was a problem.

'The following week he had the results ready for me and when I went in to see him, I could see the look of shock on his face. And, before he'd found the words to say it himself, I said, "It's cancer, isn't it?"

'The poor chap was as shocked as I was. Here I was, an apparently healthy young woman who he'd been treating for infertility and the news he now had to give me would mean I'd never be able to have a baby of my own, because I was going to need radiotherapy and a hysterectomy.

'My husband and I had been married for eight years and we'd been together ages, but, inevitably, I started to panic, wondering what on earth he'd been doing for me to develop cancer. It was, I thought, such a horribly stigmatized disease.

'But my cancer was an adenocarcinoma – the rarer type, which isn't sexually linked – and because it had been growing inwards, from the cervix into the womb, it hadn't shown up on any of the smear tests I'd had.

'Fate has a strange way of organizing our lives: if it hadn't been for the fact that I'd been wanting a baby, I never would have had the investigation which led to the cancer being discovered – and because I'd so far gone symptom-free it's possible I wouldn't be here today to tell the tale.

'My overriding concern at the news was not that I had cancer, but that I couldn't have a baby. And, rather than debilitating me, this had the effect of strengthening my resolve to get better. I decided more or less on the spur of the moment that Brian and I would have to adopt, and in order to do that I had to be completely over my illness.

'The following Sunday I started my course of internal radiotherapy – and I can't remember a thing about it. I was completely knocked out by an anaesthetic and I can honestly say, hand on heart, that I had no adverse after-effects from it.

'Two weeks later, I was readmitted to hospital for my hysterectomy, which, again, went swimmingly well. Medically, I couldn't fault the team which treated me. But, on the emotional side, they were really unable to help. And, for me and Brian, this was an extremely traumatic time. There were really horrendous episodes when we would shout and scream at each other, and I'd go into floods of tears telling Brian to find someone else who could give him children. But, overall, I realized I had to turn the trauma into something positive.

'I remember phoning friends and saying, "I've got cancer, but it's OK, I'm not going to die."

'And I felt very strongly that the only person in the world who could make me better was me. I was determined to have my family, by hook or crook, and I had to get better to do that.

'We started applying for an adoption – a major rigmarole which takes months – but, in June 1989, we eventually heard we'd been approved and should hear about our baby by Christmas.

'That summer, we spent a glorious holiday in Scotland, and I remember saying to Brian how lovely it would be to have a baby with a Scottish name.

'Christmas came and went without any news. But, then, on my birthday, 18 January, Social Services phoned to say they had a little boy called Callum for us. He had red hair (just like me!) and blue eyes, and we got him when he was just nine weeks old. Callum is now six and we are waiting for news of our second baby.

'Prior to the cancer, I was a great planner and I'd get very upset if things didn't go the way I planned. Now I take each day as it comes, and I value life much more than I ever did before.

'I also think, if it hadn't been for the cancer, I never would have known Callum – and I hate to think that he might have ended up in a situation where he wasn't as happy as he is now.

'The cancer has also had a major effect on me and Brian as a couple. I know that some couples are destroyed by illness, but for us it has had the opposite effect. Having gone through that ordeal together, we feel we can face anything.

'Sexually, it was a struggle for a long time – not because of the radiotherapy in my case, but the hysterectomy. Because I'd had a Wertheim's and had lost my ovaries, I went through an early menopause.

'I didn't feel much like sex. When we attempted intercourse, I found it very painful. And I also hated the way I looked.

'But, we've persevered and, as I am now several years into my HRT programme, things are a lot better than they were.

'And, even on the sexual side, the confrontations have forced us to talk about issues we may never have discussed before, and we are a very close and loving couple now.'

Jane Metcalfe, whom we have met at various points throughout this book, says:

> In a sense, cancer is a gift. Nothing else can scare you as much and force you to come to terms with your mortality. And I felt I had to learn to live in the present.

Jane had been told she had a 50:50 chance of dying if she didn't have the radiotherapy her oncologist recommended. But, before submitting to what she saw as a gruelling treatment, she was determined to give the holistic approach a fair chance:

> I found a more sympathetic surgeon who was happy to let me do what I wanted, and then booked myself into the Bristol Cancer Help Centre.

Before starting her course at Bristol, Jane's oncologist had given her a CAT scan to check for any rogue cancer cells.

> I didn't hear anything for six weeks, then the surgeon phoned and told me he had some bad news. The results had been lost, and, now that they'd been found, he could see something which looked like cancer. He asked me to go in so he could take another look.

By the time Jane saw him, she had received several weeks of the Bristol Cancer Help Centre's complementary therapies, and the surgeon was amazed to discover that there was absolutely no sign of the cancer that had shown up clearly on the original scan. Seven years later, there has still been no sign of the cancer returning.

> Obviously I can't say it was the complementary therapy or spiritual healing that made the cancer go away, but something happened! On the quiet, doctors admit that cancers come and go and don't always take root. I suppose that if we learn to relax, and to look after ourselves, the body is better equipped to fight them when they do appear.
>
> Cancer has certainly changed my life – in a way that is a never-ending path. I feel I am constantly moving on now. My life is not as static as it was before I became ill.

Useful addresses

The Abnormal Smear Care Helpline
Tel: 0115 9468988
For support and information after an abnormal smear.

The Bristol Cancer Help Centre
Grove House
Cornwallis Grove
Clifton
Bristol BS8 4PG
Tel: 0117–974 3216

British Pregnancy Advisory Service
Austen Manor
Wootton Wawen
Solihull
West Midlands B95 6BX
Tel: 0171 729 4688
For details of public and in-company screening programmes.

Cancerlink
17 Britannia Street
London WC1X 9JN
Tel: 0171–833 2818
For emotional support on all aspects of cancer in response to telephone and letter enquiries from people with cancer, their friends and relatives and professionals working with them.

Cercan
Tel: 0151 525 2848
For support and information following a positive smear or diagnosis of cervical cancer.

Health Information Line
Free*fone* 0800 665544
For information on all aspects of women's health, including cervical cancer, and telephone numbers and addresses of other organizations that can help.

Hysterectomy Support Network
3 Lynne Close
Green St Green
Orpington
Kent BR6 6BS
For contact with other women who have experienced hysterectomy.

National Institute of Medical Herbalists
56 Longbrook Street
Exeter EX4 6AH
Tel: 01392 462022

New Approaches to Cancer
5 Larksfield
Egham
Surrey TW20 0RB
Tel: 01784 433610
The 'nerve centre' for a network of local self-help groups, holistic practitioners and clinics throughout the UK.

Quest Cancer Test
Quest Cancer Research
Woodbury
Harlow Road
Roydon
Harlow
Essex CM19 5HF
Tel: 01279 792233
For details only of the campaign for an improved cervical screening test – they cannot offer you the test until trials have been completed.

Radiotherapy Action Group Exposure (RAGE)
24 Lockett Gardens
Trinity
Salford M3 6BJ
Tel: 0161–839 2927
For support if you have survived cancer, but are suffering severe side-effects from radiotherapy.

Transcendental Meditation (TM)
Freepost
London SW1 4YY
Tel: 0800 269303

Further reading

Chomet, Dr Jane and Chomet, Julian, *Smear Tests* (Thorsons, 1991)

Hayman, Suzie, *Hysterectomy* (Sheldon Press, 1986)

Hodgkinson, Liz and Metcalfe, Jane, *The Bristol Experience* (Vermillion, 1995)

Quilliam, Susan, *Positive Smear* (Letts, 1992)

Szarewski, Dr Anne, *A Woman's Guide to the Cervical Smear Test* (Optima, 1994)

Index